KT-173-658

WITHDRAWN

N 0029517 5

The Mind of Man

Nigel Calder

NEWMAN COLLEGE
BARTLEY GREEN
BIRMINGHAM, 32.

CLASS	*150*
ACCESSION	**22293**
AUTHOR	*CAL*

The Mind of Man

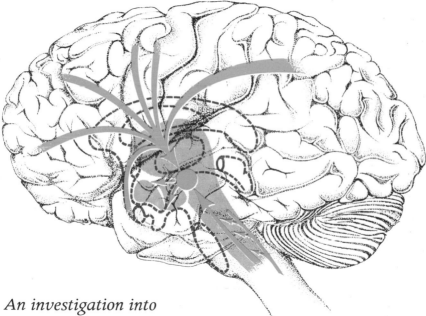

*An investigation into
current research on the brain
and human nature*

British Broadcasting Corporation

Published by the
British Broadcasting Corporation
35 Marylebone High Street
London W1M 4AA

SBN 563 10155 5

First published 1970
© Nigel Calder 1970
Printed in England by Jolly & Barber Limited,
Rugby, Warwickshire

Acknowledgment is due to the following for their permission to reproduce illustrations in this book: J. Altman, 132, 222, 223; J. S. Baily, 178; Bell Telephone Laboratories, 128; BOAC, 28; Photo Bulloz, 57; Burroughs Corporation, 273; Butterworths, 100; Camera Press, 75, 255, 277 (top); Photo CIRIC, 24; COI, 96; Annica Dahlstrom, 16 (left); Eric de Maré, 209 (top); Edinburgh University Press, 174; Daniel Farson, 209 (bottom), 212, 234; Focus (Charles Walls), 194; Fox Photos, 208; K. Fuxe, 69; R. Gregory (photo Philip Clark), 173, 180; Susan Griggs (photo Adam Woolfitt), 64; Harvard Medical School, 107; H. Hydén, 13 (top), 121; International Planned Parenthood Federation, 264; J. Jansen, 20, 21; M. Jouvet, 26; I. Kohler, 181; J. Laudenberg, 229; London Hospital, 66; Lundsuniversitets historical museum, 19; Mansell Collection, 87; D. Michie, 266–7; Josef Muench, 18; National Film Archive, 216; W. J. H. Nauta and the Neurosciences Research Program, 13 (bottom); Janet Niven, 94, 95; Popperfoto, 62, 63 (bottom), 112, 277 (bottom); Radio Times Hulton Picture Library, 89, 254; T. Rasmussen, 12; Ronan Picture Library, 157; M. R. Rosenzweig, 233; B. A. Seaby Ltd, 111; Sunday Times (Mike McInnery), 38; N. S. Sutherland, 166; Syndication International, 284; UNICEF, 218, 235; USIS, 271; H. Van der Loos, 137; William Vandivert, 129; G. von Bonin, 140; Walter Reed Army Institute of Research, 59; J. Weiss, 60; B. L. White, 231; WHO, 239.

All the remaining photographs are by Philip Daly, producer of the programme.

The poem on page 217 'A Way of Looking', by Elizabeth Jennings, is reproduced by permission of David Higham Associates.

The designer was Gerald Cinamon; the diagrams were drawn by Lynn Williams.

Author's note

The information in this book was mainly gathered in visits to laboratories of physiology and experimental psychology in eight countries during 1970, and supplemented from relevant learned papers in many different journals. The author wishes to thank the very large number of scientists who gave freely of their time and advice, including many whose work and ideas are not explicitly mentioned but who contributed to the general perspectives. The use made of the information remains the responsibility of the author.

Thanks are also due to the British Broadcasting Corporation and its associates in this project (National Educational Television, Sveriges Radio and Bayerischer Rundfunk) for the opportunity to make the world tour.

To give a complete technical bibliography would not be appropriate in a book intended for the general reader, but the following can be recommended for further reading.

For the history of psychology:
Psychology: The Science of Mental Life by G. A. Miller (Penguin Books, 1966)

For a work that helped to change the 'set' of modern psychology:
The Organization of Behavior by D. O. Hebb (Wiley, 1949)

For physiology:
The Nervous System by Peter Nathan (Penguin Books, 1969)

For general experimental psychology and physiology:
Psychobiology – readings from *Scientific American* (Freeman, 1966)

For a modern treatment of psychological research:
Cognitive Psychology by Ulric Neisser (Appleton-Century-Crofts, 1967)

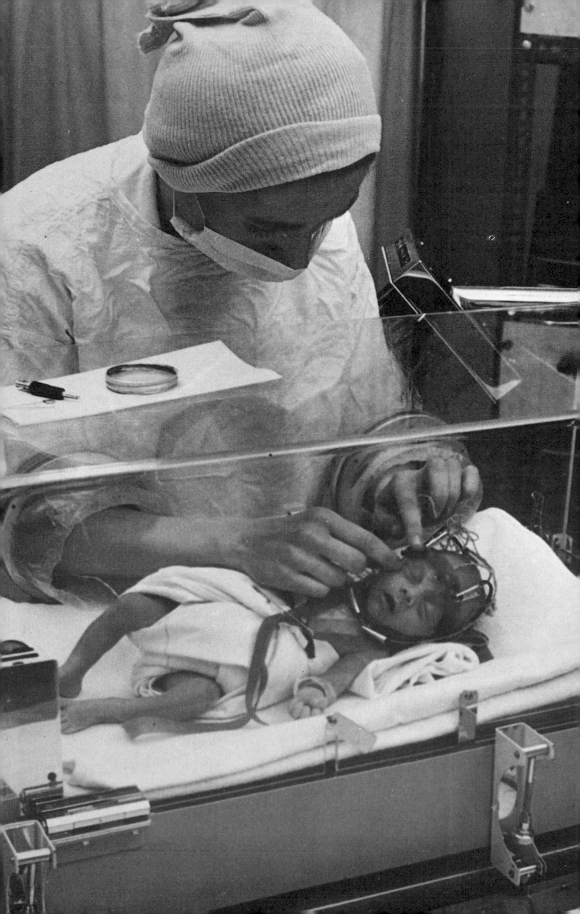

1   Nature Becomes Self-conscious

The mind of man is the very recent product of billions of years of cosmic and biological evolution and it is embodied in the most intricate of all the works of nature known to us. Can we account for human mental powers in terms of the machinery inside our heads? At least the attempt can now begin.

At a hospital in Paris, the specialists were monitoring the electrical rhythms in the head of a baby girl born prematurely. What strange fish-like dreams she might be having no one could guess; like that of other human beings born ahead of time her perception of her new environment was plainly very limited, so far. Although her legal age was already four weeks, Delphine had another five weeks to go before she would be as mature as a baby born at the right time; only then would she be ready to show some interest in the world around her.

Yet Delphine lay with the detectable rhythms of her brain testifying to the state of sleep in which older human beings, and animals too, most certainly do their dreaming. She was in the expert hands of the neo-natal research workers at the Port-Royal Maternity Hospital. She wore a crown of electric pick-

In her incubator, the premature baby Delphine discloses the tell-tale rhythms (right) of a very young mind in the making.

ups on her scalp, whence wires ran to a machine that converted waves of activity in the little brain into an agitation of pens. 'Active sleep', Nicole Monaud reported, pointing to the pattern on the moving paper, as Colette Dreyfus-Brisac looked on.

Dreyfus-Brisac has pioneered the study of brain waves in premature babies, as the first outward hints of minds in the making. Irregular flickers of electrical activity give way, as the baby grows, to more recognisable patterns, with active sleep prominent among them. These patterns of the 'electro-encephalogram', or EEG, help the doctors to assess the state of development of the child and how she should be cared for. Here is just one example of the present rapid advances in knowledge about what goes on inside the human head.

Current inquiries around the world, which are casting new light on human nature, provide the subject-matter of this book. The research and discoveries described represent only a small fraction of the recent work of the brain researchers and experimental psychologists, but I believe it is the important fraction. We are privileged onlookers during a great enlargement of knowledge and change of attitude about how the mind of man works. Barriers to understanding are collapsing, not only those due to the complexities of nature but also those created artificially by human specialisation.

Working in professional isolation, no psychologist or chemist or brain surgeon or student of animal life could show more than one facet of the brain. In the past this has led to very naive theories, doing scant justice to the powers and richness of the human mind. My very title, *The Mind of Man*, is adopted in defiance of the old convention that mind is what the psychologists deal with, in contrast with the material brain that the surgeons and physiologists handle. To a reporter taking some trouble to be objective there is plainly a movement under way, in the laboratories of several countries, which makes this distinction thoroughly out of date.

This book has been prepared simultaneously with a major television programme, filmed around the world, and owes its origin to that enterprise. In 1969 a 150-minute television programme, *The Violent Universe*, was made with the participation of the world's leading astronomers and was well received. Philip Daly as producer, and myself as writer, were asked to consider doing something on a comparable scale in another lively area of current science. We were not long in deciding that brain research was the best candidate.

Daly and I had the opportunity to go anywhere we thought necessary, looking for outstanding discoverers in brain physiology and experimental psychology. It made a fascinating

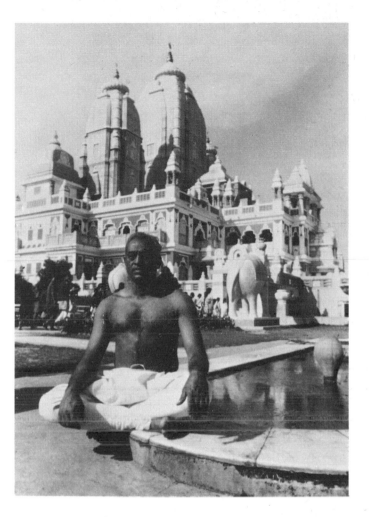

A 'raj yogi' whose powers of mind over matter have been verified by laboratory tests. In the background is the Lakshiminarain Temple, New Delhi.

journey, to meet more than a hundred experts in eight countries, each with significant things to tell about the brain. We went to New Delhi, for instance, to the laboratory where a yogi had been found capable of controlling his body in ways that were theoretically impossible. In Lyon and Edinburgh we sampled the latest opinions on sleeping and dreaming; in Munich we saw radio-controlled monkeys; in Moscow we spent many congenial hours with one of the most experienced investigators of effects of brain damage. Boston had a tight clasp on many of our topics, with Noam Chomsky's bold opinions on language showing no patience with recent orthodoxy. In Los Angeles, most thought-provoking of all, were the patients in whom brain surgery had created two separate minds inside the one head.

The enthusiastic help given to us provided fresh confirmation, if any were needed, of how anxious experimenters are that the public be kept informed of their work. There were 11 great riches for our programme. Although this book draws from the same pool of recent research it is not an adaptation of the script of the programme. The highlights are the same, but it has been separately conceived and includes information and ideas which even our two-hour programme could not accommodate.

Under the skull

The 'face barrier' is a perpetual problem for anyone to overcome who tries to imagine the brain at work. The brain seems almost like an abstract theory, even though it lies only a few millimetres behind the eyebrows. Yet it is the more durable embodiment of human and individual nature, while the face is just a kind of cinema screen across which flicker the projections of the brain's activities.

Even when exposed, human brain is not very impressive to look at. Greyish in colour and with the consistency of soft cheese, it fits snugly inside the top of the skull. It weighs about as much as a dictionary of moderate size. But this lump of tissue, your brain or mine, is the most intricate and powerful of all the works of nature known to us. It is a machine millions of times more complex than the mightiest computers now built; furthermore it is a machine that is conscious of its own existence. Here, and nowhere else, we presume, are generated the thoughts and feelings, dreams and creative actions which are the essence of human life; it is the organ of the mind of man.

The right side of a living human brain is exposed for an operation at the Montreal Neurological Institute. The numbered points show where the surgeon has given mild electrical stimulation to the surface of the brain and observed the effects on the patient, who remains conscious during the operation.

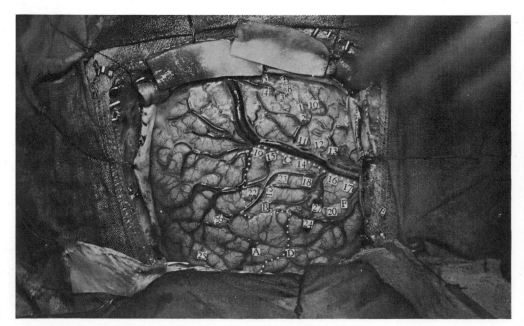

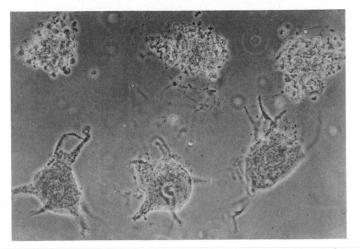

Masses of glia, or 'glue' cells (upper row), separated from the nerve cells (lower row) which they originally surrounded. (Microdissection by H. Hydén and A. Pigon)

Like all other parts of the body, and all plants and animals, the brain consists of cells, little units of life normally visible only under the microscope. There are many billions of cells in the brain. The ones most directly involved in mental and other processes are the neurons, nerve-like cells which come in many shapes and sizes and have vast numbers of connections. The others are glia, or 'glue' cells. If the cells were as big as grains of sand, they would fill a large truck. This great mass of cells is bewildering for those who try to trace its organisation and connections, but it is certainly not without pattern. The cells are arranged neatly in layers, which fact plainly has something to say about how the brain operates. Furthermore, the overall sculpture of the brain is far from meaningless.

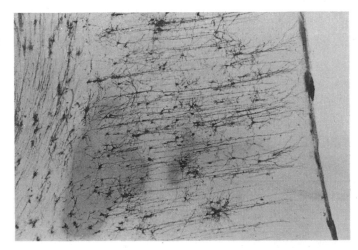

The mass of cells in the brain is not without pattern. Often they are arranged in columns and layers, as in this section of part of the cerebral cortex of a cat, where the neurons have been made visible by a staining technique. (Microphotograph by W. Nauta)

The most conspicuous part of the human brain consists of the two cerebral hemispheres on the top. The hemispheres are separated by a fissure running from front to back but they are 13 reconnected by thick cables of fibres lying towards the centre of the brain. Message-carrying fibres also fill much of the volume of the hemispheres, leaving most of the work of the brain to be done in the outermost three millimetres. This is the cerebral cortex, to which I shall often refer as 'the roof of the brain'. It is very crumpled; if it were ironed flat, it would form a sheet about half a metre square.

The upper components of the brain grow outwards from a stem. The central part of the brain, closest to the top of the brain stem, is the hub of communications for the whole brain, with busy traffic of information flowing in all directions. It also has a specialised role in the expression of drives and emotions. The brain stem itself runs down to connect with the cables of the spinal cord, whence radiates the tracery of nerves that carry signals to and from all parts of the body. The important sense organs, including those of sight, hearing and smell, have more direct access to the higher parts of the brain. At the back of the brain there is an additional component, the cerebellum, or 'little brain', which is dedicated to learning and reconstructing skilled movements.

The brain is an electrical machine. That much is evident from the EEG recorded at its outer surface, and disturbances due to epilepsy and other malfunctions appear in the wavy traces of the pen recorders. The technique was pioneered in the 1920s by Hans Berger of the University of Jena. Apart from other obvious uses in studies of sleeping, waking and excitement, the EEG recorded at the scalp remains rather disappointing. After half a century, it still tells us little about how the normal human brain works although, with modern techniques, it is possible to detect the arrival of signals in particular regions of the brain.

The intricate electric business of the brain is transacted by impulses within individual brain cells which 'fire' intermittently. These can be detected only with very fine probes, or micro-electrodes, inserted right into the brain. An understanding of the ever-changing patterns of electrical activity comes with the simultaneous tracing of connections and influences involving many individual cells, but in very few parts of the brain has this tracing been done at all thoroughly.

The brain is also a chemical machine. The discovery that chemicals are involved in nerve action outside the brain is of vintage similar to that of the EEG. In 1921 Otto Loewi of the University of Graz showed that material produced when a nerve stopped the action of one frog's heart could be used to stop the heart of another frog. The identification of chemical agents within the brain has been a slow business. But it is now

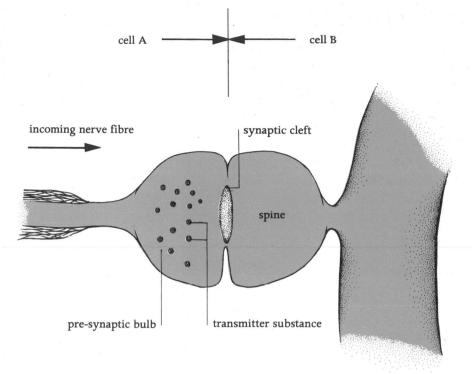

cell A   cell B

incoming nerve fibre

synaptic cleft

spine

pre-synaptic bulb

transmitter substance

The link, or synapse, between one brain cell and another. A signal travels from left to right by the release of a transmitter substance.

abundantly clear that one brain cell influences the action of another, not by direct electrical connection, but by releasing a 'transmitter' substance into a narrow gap that separates them.

Different cells use different transmitters with fairly awkward names: noradrenalin, serotonin, dopamine, GABA and acetylcholine are all now thought to figure as brain transmitters. One recent benefit of the studies of transmitters has been the introduction of dopa, a drug related to dopamine, as a treatment for many cases of Parkinson's disease. This brain disorder, which causes loss of muscular control and was known to our forefathers as the shaking palsy, is found sometimes to involve shortages of dopamine in an important mass of cells deep in the brain.

In Sweden, the transmitter business has taken on a productively vivid aspect. A group led by N. A. Hillarp, of the Karolinska Institute in Stockholm, found a way of treating slices of brain tissue in such a way that some of the transmitters would glow brightly by the light of an ultraviolet lamp. Seen under the microscope, brain cells appear bedecked with green or yellow jewels – packets of the transmitter materials. Apart from generating pictures of great beauty, this fluorescent technique makes possible important studies of how cells handle these transmitters, how chains of similar cells thread through the brain, and how the cells respond to changing circum- 15

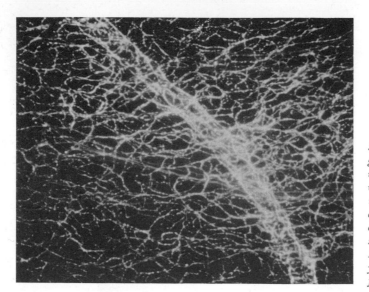

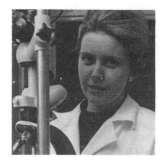

Specially treated tissue (left) glows brightly in ultra-violet light under the microscope, showing the whereabouts of transmitter material in nerve fibres in the eye of a rat. Similar networks occur in the brain but cannot be shown with equal clarity. Annica Dahlström (below) is one of the young Swedes pioneering this fluorescent technique.

stances. When Hillarp died, it fell to two of his young students, Annica Dahlström and Kjell Fuxe, to bring his work to fruition.

The big discoveries of recent years span all levels of brain structure, from the nature of the brain cells and their connections to overall organisation; and they spread across many aspects of human nature, from the primitive needs of sleeping and eating to the use of language, man's most distinctive power. Advances in other branches of science, concurrent with these discoveries, appear to be highly relevant to future explanations of the mind.

Chief among them is the great leap in knowledge about some of the basic mechanisms of life, particularly about the way the genetic material, DNA, supplies instructions in chemical code for the manufacture of particular kinds of protein, the key agents in a living system. Several of the leading molecular biologists responsible for this progress in knowledge have now switched their attention to the nervous system. In a quite different direction, mathematicians are beginning to produce theories of complex, brain-like systems which help to define possible mechanisms of learning and thinking. Closely related to such work is the attempt to supply computers or similar machines with some ability to think intelligently.

Machinery for action

The brain itself is compact enough but there is no point in regarding it as a museum-piece, isolated in a glass case. It is a working system and its structure, its contents and its affairs all depend upon interaction with events far outside it. The brain is swept by many influences and it reacts by exerting its own influence. The brain's role as servant and master of the human body ties it inseparably to the genes and all the evolution and heredity that they represent; to the fate of the body from conception to death; to the ongoing demands and ailments of the body. As the organ of experience, the brain responds and remembers its responses to the natural environment and to other people and their works. Minds make minds, from generation to generation. Finally, the brain furnishes itself with home-made experiences, in the form of ideas.

Being a product of the earth, the human brain is built of atoms that were formed in the hot interior of stars long since exploded and were sorted by cosmic distillation during the subsequent birth of the sun and its planets. On the third planet, our own, conditions were right for the sun's energy to conjure life out of the gases, water and rocks. Precisely how the first

Influences shaping the mind of man.

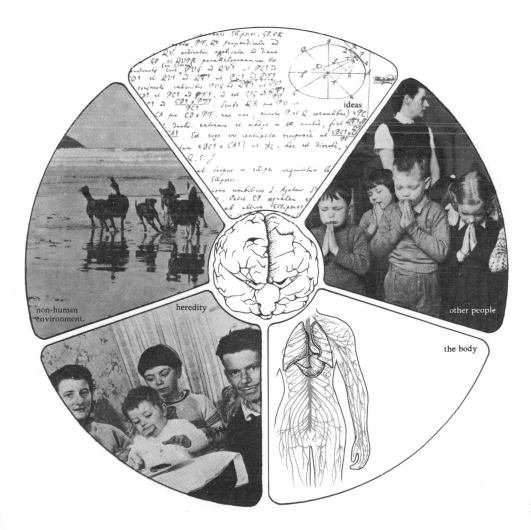

ideas

non-human
environment.

heredity

other people

the body

primitive organisms formed out of a watery soup of chemicals is still a matter of conjecture. But the chemical evidence that essential complex materials would appear spontaneously leaves no reason whatever to invoke the miraculous injection of a 'life force', or to suppose that life has not originated millions of times, on planets of other stars.

On our planet, and possibly on others, the astonishing outcome is that the collection of atoms making up living organisms have now become sophisticated enough to ask why they exist. In us, the privileged animals, nature becomes self-conscious.

Human survival and achievement are due not just to the possession of highly-developed reasoning powers, but also to the way these powers are matched to other mental faculties.

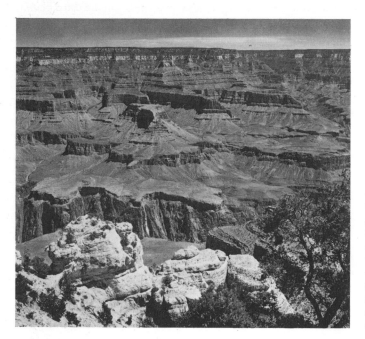

Each of these exposed layers of rock in the earth's surface represents an episode of millions of years in the slow evolution of life from primitive forms to the elaborate mammals of today. On the time-scale represented in the mighty walls of the Grand Canyon, the sojourn of man-like species on earth corresponds only to a few metres of rock, while Homo sapiens *as we know him 'appears' only in the topmost few centimetres.*

Especially important is our emotional competence. That may seem a strange phrase to use about a species that worries continually about its violence and its neuroses, but we are far more responsive and constructive in our dealings with other people that are the kindred of older species, and we have enormous capacity for endurance. The co-operation, altruism and determination that saved us when we were naked against the elements are still the basis of our present achievements.

The generosity and modesty that characterise life in the few remaining hunting tribes are a model for good conduct but we should not underestimate, either, the behavioural achievements of civilisation. In our proper concern about nationalistic and racial strife, we overlook the stable peace achieved within nations of many millions of people. The human mind is, if any-thing, too tractable and learns the ways of its teachers; also it has a great appetite for knowledge, whether of the spoor of the antelope or the physics of the atom. On top of all this, we have the gifts of tongue and hand – unique linguistic powers of com-munication and record, and unique manual powers for making an arrowhead or a transistor. These features evolved together, as mutually reinforcing qualities appropriate to a hunting animal without large teeth or claws.

They emerged with astonishing speed in about fifteen mil-lion years since our ancestors diverged from the apes. The weather probably had a lot to do with it. Before the series of Ice Ages during which modern man finally emerged, and in which we still live, the world's climate was balmy and settled. The fluctuating ice and rainfall in the past million years or so pre-sumably gave advantage to adaptable animals – and no other animal is as adaptable as man. *Homo sapiens* arrived on the scene. Since 50,000 years ago, any evolutionary changes have been quite negligible; we are essentially identical in body and mind with the Adams and Eves of the Old Stone Age.

In the intervening centuries the sages have sat down to think about thought. Good luck to them, but to do so may be thoroughly misleading. One reason is the self-deception in-volved; we can discover very little about how our minds work just by trying to sample the contents of our consciousness. Thinking about thinking about golf, say, is very different from thinking about golf and, in any case, we tend to mistake the successive products of thought for the mechanisms generating the thoughts.

There is a second reason for saying that brooding in an arm-chair can give a very false impression of the mind. Nature certainly did not select the human brain for survival, during those climatic upheavals of the Ice Ages, because of its aptitude for moral philosophy. The preoccupations of professors are by-products or bonuses of a thoroughly practical nervous system that evolved for action rather than introspection. To ignore that may be to guarantee failure in trying to grasp the principles of the brain's design. The most learned and creative human powers seem, on present evidence, to spring naturally from the highly-developed but basic skills involved in spotting an edible animal and conspiring with your mates to kill him for supper.

Even in our technological and highly-educated society human mental processes are still active rather than reflective, and the mind of man in action is wonderful to behold. The brain   19

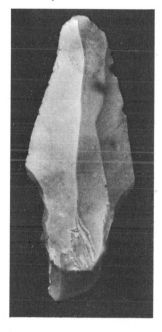

The arrowheads of our hunting forefathers testify to an aptitude for technology, one of the characteristics which favoured survival of the human brain.

of a pilot landing a big airliner is fully stretched in its powers of skill, judgement and foresight, but he thinks about his task, not about himself. The musician, the athlete and the craftsman display, in equal measure, the exquisite control of the muscles by the accomplished brain, although none may consider himself as 'brainy'. A mother talking to her child is the unassuming instrument of a formidable system of cultural evolution. If you told her she was nurturing his linguistic, manual and emotional faculties and educating him in the prevailing mores and technologies of the collective, she might laugh and say she was just trying to get Johnny to buckle his shoes.

The reader who expects much discussion of conventional psychological theories will be disappointed. Classical mental illness is seldom mentioned in this book. We shall encounter sick people, to be sure, but they will be most frequently those suffering damage to the fabric of the brain and from whom, in the efforts to treat them, medical men have learned a great deal about the workings of the brain. Even the manifest differences among individuals, in respect of personality, achieve-

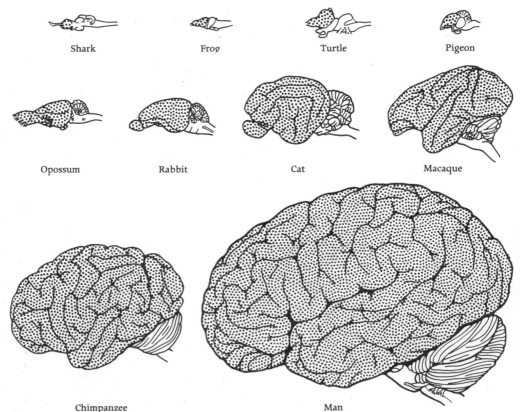

Shark Frog Turtle Pigeon

Opossum Rabbit Cat Macaque

Chimpanzee Man

ments and so forth, are dealt with only lightly. The powers of the human brain that we all share, and which distinguish all of us from any other animal, are quite enough to merit our attention.

Animal experiments

We are not wholly different from other animals. The more basic the mechanism and the longer it has been exploited in the brains of animals, the more likely it is to apply to us. Experiments with animals have to substitute for many that are unthinkable in humans. As the human brain is a thousand times bigger than the brain of a rat, the animal of choice in many experiments, thorough-going scepticism is appropriate about how we translate results from rat to man. But a man cannot be less complex than the laboratory animals.

They provide a distorting mirror of ourselves, in which we can see the true wonder of processes that are so much a part of our lives as to seem unremarkable. The present rebound

The brains of various species shown on the same scale, by Jan Jansen of the University of Oslo. Although the human brain is quite big, it is small in bulk compared with that of one of the smallest whales.

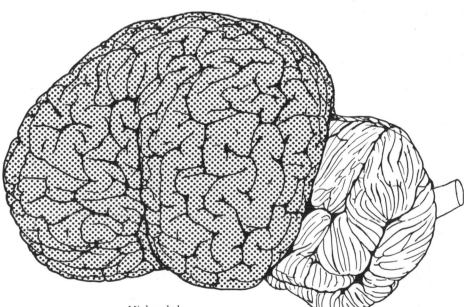

Minke whale

21

from oversimplified theories is due in part to the fact that they cannot fully account even for the performance of experimental animals, starting with the Harvard law of animal behaviour: 'When the same stimulus is given repeatedly under carefully controlled conditions the animal will behave as it damned well pleases'.

The human brain is three times bigger even than a chimpanzee's brain, although it contains only one quarter more of the active brain cells, the neurons. Brain size is in any case a very crude measure of the likely abilities of a brain. Elephants and whales, with much bigger brains than ours, are far from stupid but they give no sign that they are cleverer than we are, in any respect.

Remarks of a different kind are necessary about the animal experiments we shall consider. A bystander would be insensitive not to grieve for the caged laboratory animals who pay with their emotions and their lives for the knowledge that we humans gain from them. As to what is ethical, everyone would draw his own line, somewhere between teaching a dog to beg and major surgery without an anaesthetic. One or two of the experiments mentioned in the book fall beyond what I should ever have a hand in. But in nearly all vivisection careful surgery and ample anaesthesia eliminate pain.

Brain tissue itself is incapable of pain. This point, which led Aristotle to deny that the brain could be the seat of feelings, is worth keeping in mind when we come across animals (and humans) whose brains are modified with the surgeon's knife or with implanted electrodes. In some other experiments, fully conscious animals receive electric shocks unless they learn to avoid them. An apparatus for such purposes was described by an experimental psychologist as a 'torture chamber'. One of his colleagues thereupon built a bridge from home cage to shock box and found that an experienced mouse would run spontaneously into the 'torture chamber' and wait for the trials.

Finally, medicine supplies the ultimate justification for most animal experiments – which are by no means confined to brain studies, of course. There can be scarcely anyone in an industrialised country who has not benefited medically from animals and the relief of human mental suffering due to animal experiments is already incalculable.

Mind and brain

The aim in the pages that follow is to see how far we can go in explaining, in terms of brain mechanisms, the human mental powers of which we are all aware. Some of the endless quibbling about the meaning of the term 'mind', as opposed to the term 'brain', will have to be made explicit near the end of the book, especially in considering consciousness. Meanwhile I wish only to take as a working assumption the idea that the mind and the brain are inseparable, and to put it no more strongly or precisely. The mind is often said to comprise the contents or operations of the brain. As mental operations seem to alter the fabric of the brain, it may be nearer the mark to say the mind *is* the brain.

The verbal formula is much less important than the practical question of how the brain makes possible the various ingredients of mental life such as seeing and acting, remembering and thinking. Although it is down to earth, this question is not a modest one. It implies an attempt to bring the human conscious mind back into the physical world, whence it was ejected by René Descartes in 1637. He drove it out for the best of motives, so that it could be immortal. But now that heaven and hell are out of fashion, the mind of man has been left impotently in limbo.

In recounting the discoveries and ideas of the new era in brain research, I shall be accused of wanting to reduce the marvels of man's mind to 'nothing but' electrical and chemical processes in brain tissue, in short of 'reductionism'. But that term is just one among several, like 'mentalism' and 'dualism', which tend to be used as landmines to prevent an argument proceeding along unwelcome lines. The attempt to account for our mental life by reference to the brain is rejected by some as leaden and futile. Whether futile, only time will tell; but whether leaden depends on the strategy. Psychological facts and impressions have to be explained, not by oversimplifying them to conform with what we know about the brain, but by enlarging our knowledge of the brain to accommodate them. As a distinguished Canadian psychologist, Donald Hebb, would put it, this is not degrading mind to matter. Instead, it is upgrading the properties of matter to account for mind.

The philosophical questions are, in any case, too important to be left to the philosophers; also too urgent, for two kinds of reasons. A radical change in human ambitions is in prospect, as our social structures creak under the new technologies, the threat of instant annihilation and the semi-articulate discontents of both rich and poor peoples; any reappraisal of social aims requires the best possible understanding of human nature.

Secondly, there are more direct consequences of brain research. Drugs that have very powerful effects on the mind and are being widely misused supply the most obvious current

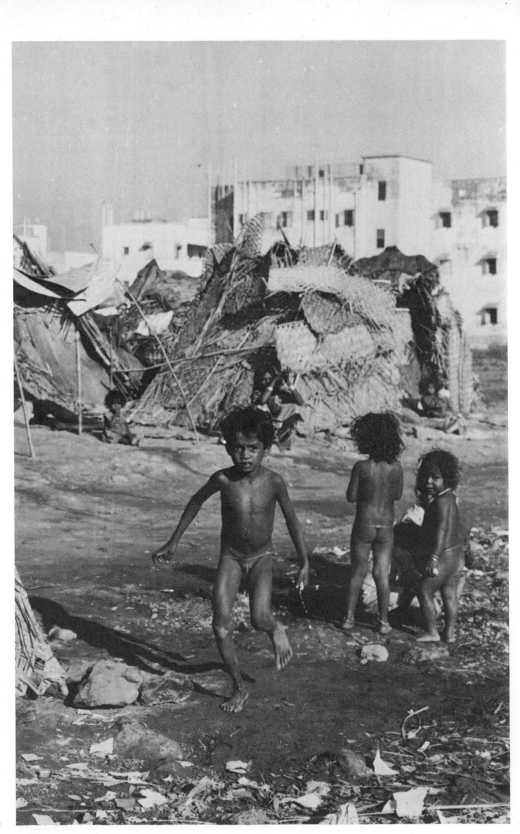

example. As a hint of possibilities to come, Robert White, a surgeon in Cleveland, Ohio, experiments in the transplantation of the brains of animals. He can keep them alive, either naked on the bench or embedded in the body of another animal. Although reconnection of a brain to the nerves of the body is technically impossible at present, White speculates about eventual extension of human mental life by brain transplants. Whether we should ever tolerate such procedures would depend upon our views on the relation of mind and body, and on human values.

Exploration of the brain, in search of the recognisable qualities of the human mind, will naturally involve us in many questions of everyday life, about sexuality and emotion as well as about our intellectual powers. Topics along the way include the subjectivity of sight, the organisation of foresight, and the fashion in which the successive achievements of a child match the gradual completion of his brain. Encouragingly often there will be concrete evidence about the location and methods of operation of machinery within the brain. At other times we must use our imagination to persuade ourselves that there is nothing about our imaginations that cannot ultimately be related to the firing of cells in the brain.

Two of the most self-evident characteristics of the conscious mind show at once a contrast in the state of knowledge about the brain mechanisms involved. One is the fact that the mind attends to one thing at a time, to produce a series of thoughts and considered actions, rather than striving to deal with everything at once. For this guiding principle of our mental life the machinery can only be guessed at. On the other hand, a second feature of the conscious mind is that, at least once a day, it is switched off. The discovery of where that happens is one of the achievements of recent brain research.

Improved understanding of human nature, from brain research, should help to define the ill-effects of social neglect, especially in children, like these young Indians.

EEG

neck muscle

eye movement

neck more relaxed

onset of rapid eye movements

cat goes into REM sleep

2 The Master Switches

*The mind directs its attention to one main interest at a time
but it craves continuous and varied excitement. The
mechanisms of waking, sleeping and dreaming are now being
thoroughly explored and recordings of eye movements
have already transformed our knowledge of when people dream.*

A cat starts dreaming, as shown by the pens of a recorder at the Lyon School of Medicine.

A sailor of the Royal Navy sat in a darkened room far from sea, at Cambridge, a little lightheaded after a big swig of rum, playing a game for the psychologists. To add to his problems, a loudspeaker filled the room with noise. He sat at a table operating some simple controls. He had to track an erratically-moving needle by shifting a handle with his right hand; he was also required to respond to 'warning signals' shown by a spread of lights by pressing corresponding switches with his left hand. The sailor performed the basic task as well as he would have done in peace and sobriety, if not better. But the experiment was so arranged that one of the warning lights came on only rarely, and that one he tended to miss.

The sailor was concentrating on his task and ignoring the distractions. That was normal enough, but the noise and the alcohol and his emotional state combined to make him concentrate on watching for the more frequent signals. Peter Hamilton, who was running the test, noted that either the sailor overlooked the unexpected light or else his reaction was hesitant, as if he needed more evidence before believing what he did not expect to see. The effect of all the stress was not distracting in the normal sense but rather the reverse; the sailor's attention was narrowed.

This situation was typical of the work of the British government's Applied Psychology Research Unit at Cambridge, which is called on for practical advice about watch-keeping in ships, shift work in factories, the mistakes made by car drivers and pilots, and the best ways of displaying information. Almost anyone would respond like the sailor in this kind of stressful situation, missing the unexpected. In real life, the consequences of oversight can be very grave. But although their

27

work has these eminently practical aspects, the experimenters in this research unit find themselves continually dealing with fundamental issues about the way the brain works and having to evolve theories of mental mechanisms to account for these everyday features of human behaviour.

'Attention is the bit of machinery which decides from moment to moment what it is we're going to notice and therefore what we shall do.' Thus does Donald Broadbent, director of the Cambridge unit, put one of the fundamental issues in the plainest terms. 'None of us can take in at the same time everything that is striking our eyes and our ears. There seems to be a kind of filter inside the head which protects the central systems against being overloaded.'

With carefully-designed experiments, psychologists can test some of the features of the machinery of attention. In early work Broadbent concluded that it took about a sixth of a

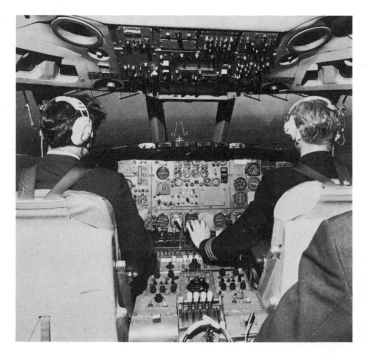

Landing an aircraft at night. The effect of stress is to make a man concentrate very narrowly on the task in hand.

Donald Broadbent : 'There seems to be a kind of filter inside the head.'

second to redirect attention, as from one ear to the other, but a man could normally make the switch no more often than about once a second. Anne Triesman of Oxford University is one of the investigators who have sought to extend and modify Broadbent's basic description of attention as a filter protecting the 'central systems' from an excess of information. It seems that the rate at which information is registered in our minds is not precisely limited, because we can understand something said to us even at twice the normal speed.

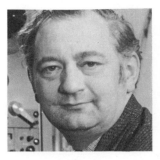

The possible strategies whereby the brain selects what it shall attend to, and what it will do about it, are varied, a little complex, and incompletely tested. They include: concentration on a particular feature, as when looking for misprints, for example; concentration on particular people or objects; and looking for information relevant to a particular goal. Triesman also emphasises the difference between two kinds of situation. One is where we try to focus attention on one thing, and exclude distractions – that is an efficient process in humans. On the other hand, dividing attention between two or more matters of interest is possible only if there is time to switch attention back and forth. Evidently we can think clearly only about one set of information at one instant.

However sharply we focus our attention, and cut out distractions, part of the brain is always vigilant. Some events will rouse the mind from its reverie because they are startling; if someone now came through the door with a gun in his hand, you would not continue dutifully to the end of this sentence. Milder signals can be very effective if they are important and half-expected. A mother may sleep through a bombardment yet wake promptly when the faint cries of her baby reach her ears – unless she happens to be dreaming. A man may ignore the background hubbub at a party, until someone across the room mentions his name.

So the filter of attention, if there is such a thing, cannot be a complete block to background information. Triesman has suggested that the filter can only weaken the unwanted signals, leaving them available to other brain mechanisms to seize upon if necessary. But a quite different possibility is that the focusing of attention is an inherent part of the mechanisms of seeing or listening. If so, the incoming information is not shut out from the brain or weakened; it is simply not analysed. This is the view of Ulric Neisser, of Cornell University, and we shall meet it again in other contexts.

In any case, no one can yet pinpoint with confidence the sites of these theoretical machines in the brain. Attention is plainly one of the most important aspects of human mental operations that remain to be explained in the years ahead, before we can tell precisely how that sailor at Cambridge came to overlook a plainly visible light. One part of the brain is known to be actively involved in the management of attention (the brain-stem net, to which we shall turn in a moment), but that bit of geography does not explain how the decisions of attention are made. After a long and successful career spent locating very specific functions within the brain, Wilder Penfield, of the Montreal Neurological Institute, has said: 'If I had another life to devote to human neurophysiology, I would like to devote it to the neuronal mechanism that makes possible the focusing of attention.'

A network for arousal

To try to rank the departments of the brain in order of importance is a little absurd, because all play their part in normal life. Nevertheless, there has for long been a tendency to regard the roof of the brain, the cerebral cortex, as the highest region, hierarchically as well as anatomically. It is, after all, the seat of rational thought and its great size in man helps to distinguish us from other animals. But such a rating undervalues the role of the brain as the great integrator of the human being in action. The modern view is more democratic.

If the primary job of the brain is to enable its owner to respond effectively to events, the strongest claimant for mastery is not the roof at all, but the brain stem. This is the stalk-like mass of cells running from the top of the spine into the very middle of the brain. In evolutionary terms it is an old and primitive part of the brain. But it exerts its authority most conspicuously every time we fall asleep, or wake up.

The core of the brain stem contains a fine net of interconnected cells, the 'reticular formation' in anatomist's jargon. This brain-stem net, no bigger than your little finger, is well placed to monitor all the nerves connecting brain and body. It 'knows' what is going on better than any other single part of the brain. In its exercise of overall control, it disdains detail. The brain-stem net is concerned with the overall pattern of activity and with inspiring greater effort in various sectors of the brain and the outlying nervous system, as required. A single cell in the net may receive impulses from an astonishing variety of sources.

In a paper in *The Neurosciences*, Madge and Arnold Scheibel of the University of California, Los Angeles, have described the action of the net at the core of the brain stem as follows:

> Competition for the interest of the reticular arrays must be high, and supremacy is gained for the moment in time only by those data that are most 'exotic' — or most compelling biologically. Like some stern, harried father figure, the core has limited patience and limited time-binding resources. Its logic is wide but superficial and its decisionary apparatus does not permit the luxury of hesitation.

The brain-stem net exerts its authority by sending out impulses which stimulate or inhibit nerve action throughout the

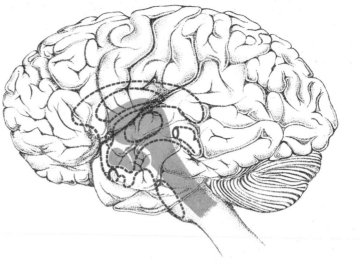

The brain-stem net (shaded area) extends into the central regions of the brain. The lower part provides the 'reticular activating system' which is responsible for arousal and wakefulness. (After Livingston)

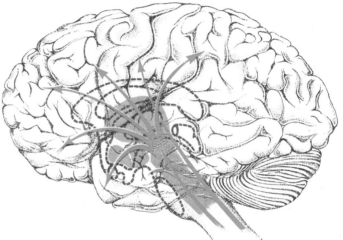

An impression of how the brain-stem net influences much of the rest of the brain, to sustain general activity. (After Magoun)

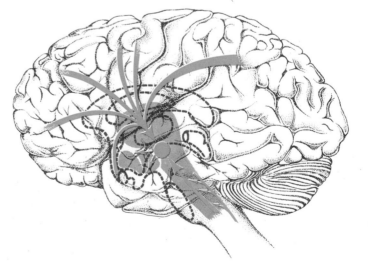

Commands from the upper and central regions of the brain converge with sensory signals in the brain stem and the activating net is informed of what is going on. (After Livingston).

brain and body. It can override activity in the spinal cord, the great cable of nerves running up the back. It regulates the signals from the eyes, ears and other sense organs, thereby providing, as already mentioned, an agency for selecting what is to be attended to, from moment to moment.

Although suspicions about the importance of the stem net had been growing from several decades previously, decisive evidence came in 1949 when Giuseppe Moruzzi and Horace Magoun (then at Northwestern University, Illinois) showed that signals from the brain stem are necessary for keeping the roof of the brain awake and active. Subsequently, it has turned out that sleeping, too, depends on positive actions by the brain stem – not just on a relaxation of the 'wake-up' signals.

At just about the same time as the Magoun – Moruzzi discovery of the 'reticular activating system' of the brain-stem net, there was published the most important of recent attempts at a comprehensive theory of the brain in action : *The Organization of Behavior*, by Donald Hebb of Montreal. Twenty years later Hebb, who is now chancellor of McGill University, says his theory cannot possibly be completely right – indeed there are points in it which have already turned out to be wrong – but he is very content with the way in which several of the key ideas are being borne out by new experimental results.

His objective was the same as ours, to explain the human mind in terms of brain mechanisms, without any supernatural or other extraneous factors. Hebb was of course working at the level of scientific originality, while I am just a reporter. His ideas of 1949 and after will crop up in various chapters of this book. But one of the areas in which Hebb's theory matured most rapidly, in the 1950s, concerns our present interest in arousal and levels of consciousness. In his book, he suggested that, with insufficient information coming from the senses, the brain might become emotionally disturbed. In this, he was quickly proved to be correct.

Some of Hebb's students at McGill (Woodburn Heron and others) undertook to investigate what happens to a human brain which is largely deprived of input from the senses. Apart from the theoretical interest of the question, the ill-effects of boredom at work, in hospital, and in solitary confinement, are matters of practical concern. It was not practicable to deprive each paid volunteer of all sensation, but anything conveying patterns or organised information was denied to him as far as was possible. He lay on a bed with his ears blocked, his hands wrapped in gloves and big cardboard cuffs, and a translucent visor over his eyes.

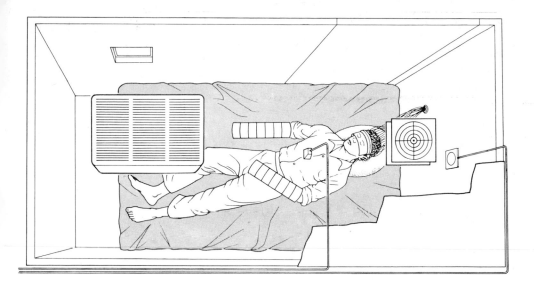

Without information from the out-side world, the brain becomes inefficient and liable to hallucina-tions. This is how volunteers were dressed for experiments in 'sensory deprivation' at McGill University. (After Heron)

Although the volunteers were healthy, impecunious college students, who received twenty dollars a day just to do nothing, some of them gave up on the first day. Those who could stand it for longer were strangely affected by the experience. They had hallucinations. sights of marching squirrels, parades of eyeglasses, sounds of a music box or a church choir. After four days, they found that the world seemed distorted and that their power to do simple tests was impaired for a while.

The results of these and many subsequent experiments in sensory deprivation give clear evidence that the human brain depends, for its normal alertness, reliability and efficiency, on a continuous inflow of information about the world. They fit in well with the idea of curiosity. The brain craves for informa-tion as the body craves for food, and other animals besides men will go to some pains to see new sights. Man's nearest relatives, the apes and monkeys, are especially inquisitive.

Hebb himself knew all about the human need for something interesting to do. He had once carried out, with confidence and complete success, a radical educational experiment which is not so well known as it should be. All of the 600 pupils in a school were punished by being sent out to play and were per-mitted to work as a reward for being good. Within a couple of days, teaching at that school was proceeding more efficiently and with better discipline than ever before, because the child-ren preferred arithmetic to boredom.

In a revised presentation of ideas, in 1955, relating arousal, attention and emotion, Donald Hebb drew the diagram shown overleaf. It is only schematic – there are no measures on the

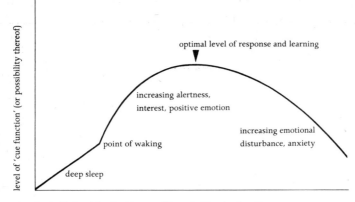

Donald Hebb's diagram suggesting that a certain amount of excitement ('arousal function') is necessary for the brain to be efficient but that excessive excitement or emotional disturbance reduces efficiency. The 'cue function' of the vertical scale denotes the practical response of the brain to an incoming signal.

graph – but it conveys, more readily than words, the idea that mild excitement is necessary for the brain to work at its most efficient; also that when the arousal becomes intense emotion the efficiency falls off sharply. The expressions 'blind with rage' and 'rigid with fear' are not fanciful, while a person exposed to more trouble than he can cope with may simply fall asleep.

The commonplace observation that some people are more quickly overtaken by boredom than others seems to fit in with the new ideas about the brain, and to supply the first strong link between normal brain mechanisms and differences of human personality. The distinction between introverts and extroverts is one of long standing. It divides people (along a continuous scale, not into sharply-defined groups) into those who are sociable, impulsive, easy-going and quick-tempered on the one hand, and those who are retiring, calculating, serious and unaggressive on the other. Some brain researchers now reason that an extrovert is simply a person whose brain is less easily aroused than the introvert's and whose brain stem therefore needs a stronger sensory input to keep it active. An introvert, on the other hand, is more easily disturbed and made anxious by excitement.

But everyone needs stimulation. The elaborate games and sports that humans organise for themselves are often far from pleasurable in any simple meaning of that word, if one judges by the subdued anger of the bridge table, the football field or the cockpit of a yacht. Quite sensible people will risk their lives on a mountainside or on a motor-cycle rather than be bored, and war is unfortunately one of the most interesting games that man has invented. The arousal system of the brain probably holds more illuminating explanations of human conduct than does the recent emphasis on sexual and aggressive drives.

Even disagreeable treatment is better than total neglect and blandness in the environment. This was shown very strikingly in infant rats, in the mid-1950s. Seymour Levine, then at Ohio State University, decided to see what effects mild electric shocks, given daily, had upon the development of the rats. To his surprise, instead of ill-effects appearing in the rats so treated, it was another group of rats, kept for comparison without any handling in infancy, who were emotionally disturbed when he came to test them. Rats which were shocked or handled had learned to cope with stress with a quick production of appropriate hormones; the unhandled rats had not.

Sleeping and waking

At the School of Medicine at Lyon a cat was fast asleep, the time being noon and, according to Michel Jouvet, a customary hour for the cats of Europe to sleep and dream. A second cat, though, was wide awake, because he had been dosed with the 'pep' drug, amphetamine. More surprisingly, the sleeping cat had received the same dose of the drug. How was he able to sleep in spite of it?

As Jouvet explained, the sleeping cat had received, six hours earlier, another drug which cut his brain's supply of a natural transmitter chemical, noradrenalin. That material normally serves as the means of communication between some of the brain cells. But without it, a strong dose of amphetamine was no deterrent to sleep. Noradrenalin seems to be essential for the normal waking state, as nature's own 'pep' drug. Using the Swedish technique for making the brain's chemical transmitters glow in ultraviolet light, Jouvet could show the characteristic green fluorescence of noradrenalin, in the critical region of the brain stem.

Jouvet is one of the leaders of the research which has completely transformed our understanding of the main states of the brain – waking, light sleep, and the so-called 'paradoxical sleep', where dreaming is most vivid. All require special action to produce them, each having identifiable switches in the stem of the brain. As we have seen, the 'reticular activating system' of the brain-stem net is necessary for alert wakefulness. A quite separate mechanism is required for normal sleep, based on the so-called raphe system lying along the axis of the brain stem, behind the activating system. Brain cells employing another transmitter chemical, serotonin, come into prominence in the sleeping brain. If the raphe system is des-

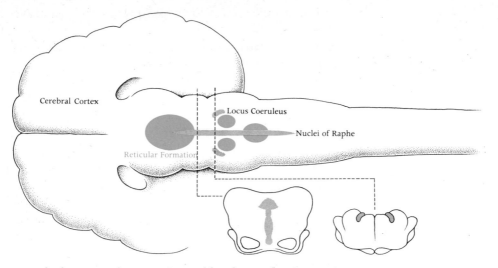

Cerebral Cortex

Locus Coeruleus

Nuclei of Raphe

Reticular Formation

troyed, the owner becomes incapable of ever sleeping again, however tired he may be.

For dreaming sleep, yet another region, the so-called locus coeruleus, also in the brain stem, has to come into play. Whatever is going on in the dream, the dreamer should not act it out by rising from his bed and rushing around. That requirement is also met by the switching machinery in the brain stem and, if it is damaged in a cat, the animal will be seen catching imaginary mice in his sleep. Conversely, the dreaming mechanism should not be switched on during waking hours. William Dement of Stanford University has suggested that the waking delusions of mental illness may in fact be due to just a slight malfunction of this specific brain process. Similar effects occur in normal people deprived of sleep.

The regularity of sleeping and waking depends on a built-in 'biological clock' in the brain, the resetting of which is a perpetual problem for long-distance air travellers. The very precise timekeeping which allows some sleepers to wake up at a chosen time without the aid of an alarm clock cannot yet be explained, but the overall cycle of sleeping and waking seems to be at least partly in the charge of the pineal gland. This is a pea-like gland behind the brain stem, which René Descartes regarded as the chosen residence of the human soul. In frogs, the equivalent organ serves as a third eye, in the top of the head, detecting through the skin the daily changes of light and darkness. In humans, the pineal gland is buried too deeply to work in that fashion, but it does receive information indirectly from the eyes. It appears to respond to darkness by producing a hormone, melatonin, which in turn influences the brain cells that use serotonin – the chemical transmitter already noted as being involved in sleep mechanisms.

The brain stem of a cat, showing switches of waking (reticular formation), sleeping (raphe nuclei) and dreaming (locus coeruleus). (After Jouvet).

The way a human being slumps under the force of gravity, fidgets on his back or side until he finds a comfortable position, and falls asleep is so familiar and welcome a transition that we usually think nothing of it. But anyone who has struggled as a sentry or night driver or nurse to keep awake when the tide of sleep rises in the brain, knows how insistent is nature's demand that this change should occur. Most adults can skip one full night's sleep, but a second is hard to endure and after a third sleepless night we may find ourselves having dream-like hallucinations. Even fear of death or punishment may be scarcely enough to suppress sleep. Sooner or later, sleep fells us, as surely as a blow on the head, and makes us apparently unconscious of our surroundings.

But most normal sleep is not at all like a knock-out (or a coma or a drunken stupor) even though these states may appear the same at a casual glance. The most obvious difference is that the sleeper retains the ability to wake 'with a start' in response to a word, a touch, a smell of smoke. And this is one clue that sleeping is only approximately a condition of unconsciousness. Another clue is the way a person changes positions repeatedly during sleep; a third is dreaming and a fourth is the fact that many cells of the brain are more active at night than in the day.

A person typically spends in sleep the equivalent of more than twenty years of his life, more time in fact than he spends learning or working or enjoying himself. In the traditional view, sleep is a mere absence of consciousness, a waste of time, a kind of daily death. Even in recent years, distinguished scientists have speculated about abolishing sleep, perhaps by suitable drugs, so that our effective living time can be increased by a third. But research workers who examine sleep itself form a much more positive view of its role in life. This role goes well beyond mere bodily rest or relief from the mental cares of waking life.

The electric rhythms of the brain, those gross indicators of brain activity in the EEG, change as a person falls asleep, but certainly do not cease. The maximum electric activity now occurs at the front of the head, rather than at the back. The rhythmic or jagged pattern of the waking state is replaced by other rhythms. In 1958, when William Dement was at the University of Chicago, he discovered alternating periods of high-voltage, slow beat, and low-voltage, fast beat, in the electric rhythms of sleeping cats.

Dement at first called the fast-beat phase 'light sleep', but in fact this rapid electrical beat turned out to be associated with the deeper periods of sleep. Jouvet, in Lyon, chose the phrase 'paradoxical sleep', because of the apparent contradiction 37 between the fast electric activity and the difficulty of arousing the sleeper. Since then, the explanation of the paradox has become apparent: the brain is otherwise engaged, in busy dreams.

Why dream?

Even as you are dropping off to sleep, hallucinations occur – a meaningless but graphic sequence of images flicker through the conscious like a series of slides, and sometimes there are feelings of floating that end abruptly in an imagined fall. These hallucinations are a foretaste of the strange mental world we inhabit in our sleep. From Joseph and the Pharaoh to Sigmund

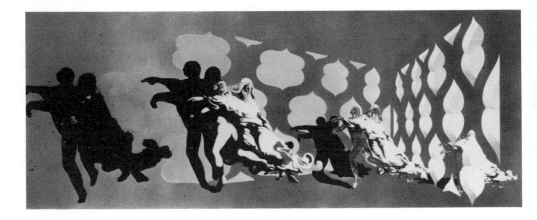

Freud, there is a long history of men trying to understand the meaning of their own and others' dreams. But it is only in the past fifteen years or so that the act of dreaming has become open to objective study. The big step forward came in the mid-1950s, after Nathaniel Kleitman and his colleagues at the University of Chicago stumbled upon an easy method of recording eye movements during sleep.

That people jerked their eyeballs when dreaming, as if looking about them in their dreams, had long been suspected. The present era of dream research began when electric pick-up leads were attached to the skin on either side of a person's eye, and connected to the pen-recorder on an EEG machine. Electric signals associated with eye movements gave a ready indication of periods of rapid eye movements, or REMs for short, even while the sleeper was left undisturbed in the dark.

By waking sleepers during REMs, the experimenters quickly established that they almost invariably said they were dreaming. If woken from sleep when REMs were not occurring, the sleepers seldom had any vivid dreams to report. In short,

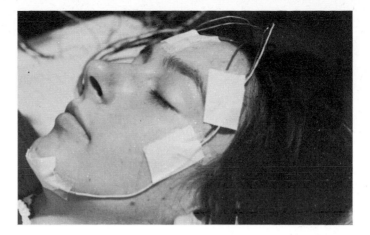

A girl volunteer sleeps and dreams for the psychiatrists at Edinburgh University. Detectors beside the eye, for recording the rapid eye movements, have transformed our knowledge of when and how much we dream.

REMs are a fairly reliable signal that the sleeper is dreaming, although milder streams of ideas seem to continue at other times of the night.

Almost immediately, REM research disposed of a lot of folklore about dreaming. On the basis of misleading subjective impressions, ordinary people and psychologists in the past spoke of 'dreamless nights' or else of 'dreaming all night'. Another favourite idea was that dreams were remarkably compressed – elaborate sequences of events being experienced by the dreamer in a few seconds. These notions have been falsified by REM research. Every healthy person dreams for several periods every night, whether or not he remembers doing so when he wakes. Moreover, events in dreams occur at roughly the same rate as they would in real life.

If I can use 'dreaming' as a shorthand for the vivid experiences of REM sleep, the night's total of dreaming is altogether an hour or two, in three to five episodes. In a typical case, at the start of the night's sleep, a person first falls into deep, undisturbed sleep. After about an hour, about ten minutes' dreaming occurs. Then there is another lull, of an

Dreaming occurs in a number of episodes through the night, as in this typical case. (After Dement)

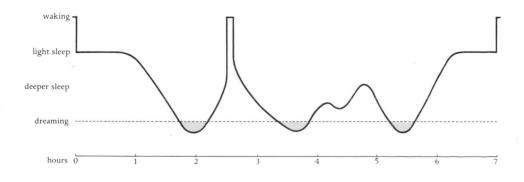

hour or more, followed by a longer period of dreaming. Through the night, the alternation of dreaming and no-dreaming continues, the dreaming periods becoming longer towards morning.

Dreams are best recalled immediately on waking. After a few minutes they may be completely forgotten unless they were particularly exciting or nightmarish. This has been a serious disadvantage for psychoanalysts and others who attach importance to the contents of dreams. Now that the psychologist can tell by the REM technique when a person is dreaming, he can wake him up and obtain a much fresher and more reliable account of dreams than is possible next morning. When a patient goes to his analyst, he may tell the dreams very differently from the way he reported them during the night, to the REM man.

But why do we dream? Clear evidence that ordinary, non-REM sleep is a period when the body is being repaired came in 1968–9 from Japanese and American work showing that, during this stage of sleep, a hormone is released which is responsible for bodily growth. According to Ian Oswald of Edinburgh University, the dreaming periods of sleep are allocated to the repair of the tissue of the brain itself. That may well be so and it fits nicely with the fact that babies sleep and dream so much when their brains are growing rapidly.

But it still gives little clue as to why the process should involve bizarre imaginings in which the events of the previous day may be mixed up, in story form, with all kinds of extraneous elements. When we went to Oswald's sleep laboratory, to waken a girl who was obligingly dreaming for us, she reported two pirates with bicycles, who were crashing them together. As dreams go, it was ordinary enough and, up to a point, it was understandable because the girl herself had been in a cycling accident the day before. But why pirates? Those who regret the intrusion of science into human mental processes may find comfort in such unexplained creativity.

Although the reason for dreams eludes us, the patterns of dreaming are very revealing. One of the most important phenomena currently engaging the interest of researchers in the USA and Britain is the rebound effect – the fact that if a person is prevented from dreaming for a period, he will thereafter spend much more time dreaming than a normal person does during his sleep. It is as if the brain were making up for lost dreams. One of the ways in which dreaming is unwittingly reduced is by sleeping pills, and this raises the awkward question of whether doctors, in prescribing barbiturates, have

40 been denying their patients restoration of the brain.

How necessary the dreaming periods are, for normal mental life, is uncertain. A famous experiment of Dement's suggested that, if volunteers were woken up every time they started to dream, they became anxious or irritable and suffered hallucinations during the day. But these results have not really been borne out in subsequent studies. What seems more definite is that appetite and sexuality are increased by loss of dreaming. The 'rebound' effect usually shows very clearly when dream-deprived people have the chance to sleep normally, but Vincent Zarcone and his colleagues at Stanford University found that it did not occur in schizophrenic patients. It was as if they had enough dreaming while awake. This is one of the reasons that led Dement to his suggestion of a defect in the switching arrangements in mental illness.

The irregularities of heart and breath that accompany dreaming suggest an ascendency of emotion. Oswald thinks that the cycle of light and sleep and dreaming is continued in recurring periods through the waking day. He has evidence, possibly inadequate so far, that covert urges become particularly important at 90-minute intervals through the day. People may then be more likely to nibble a snack, take a drink, finger their mouths and noses, and to feel sexually aroused, than at other times.

These are just a few examples from recent studies of dreaming. Uncertainties and disagreements remain about the facts of dreaming and their interpretation, but the investigators are plainly coming near to a very comprehensive account of this ingredient of our mental life and of the brain mechanisms that produce it. Already we can glimpse unsuspected aspects of human nature, not only of the night but the day as well.

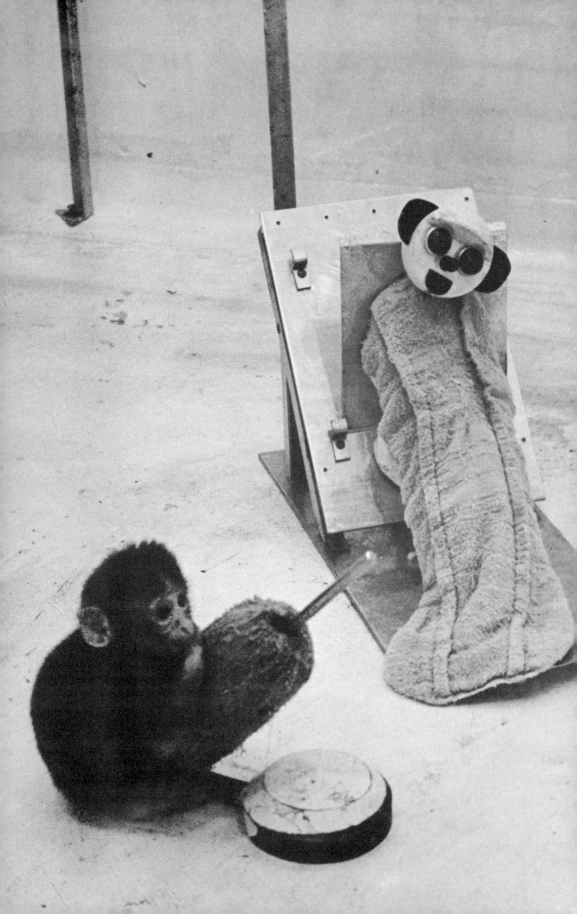

Sex and Love

Central sites in the brain organise simple drives, including sex,
while love and other complex emotions involve larger regions.
The emotions are instruments of social life, as experiments with
monkeys confirm. Contrary to recent belief, men and
women are born with markedly different emotional tendencies.

A young monkey which has grown up with the simple cloth-covered stand in place of a mother. He prefers it to the more lifelike 'mother' in the same cage.

Two female laboratory rats were brought together in a cage at Stanford University, to demonstrate the remarkable condition of one of them. This rat promptly approached the other female and she went through all the motions of copulation, as if she were a male. It was no momentary aberration of the kind that female animals sometimes show. The experimenter, Seymour Levine, had predicted this performance, because the rat in question was transexual.

When she was newborn, at a critical stage in the development of her brain, the rat had been given an injection of a male sex hormone, testosterone. The single injection was sufficient to alter her for life. Levine can make rats sexually mixed up, at will. In 1965 he was one of a group led by Geoffrey Harris, at the Institute of Psychiatry in London, which first reported firm evidence that sexuality is built into the brain. It is not just shaped by emotional experience and sustained by the trickle of hormones from the sexual glands. Male and female brains are different.

The ovaries of the masculinised female fail to mature and she generally conducts herself like a male. A male mouse castrated at birth, and therefore deprived of sex hormone at the same critical stage of brain development, goes through life as a female; as an adult he will respond like a female to a shot of female sex hormone. Injections of the 'wrong' hormone into normal adult rats produce only mildly transexual behaviour.

Manhood has to assert itself, in the normal development of the male brain. The tendency in mammals is such that if nothing intervenes, in the form of male hormone, the brain will be female. In rats, the critical period when the brain 'decides' whether it is male or female occurs in the first four

43

days after birth, but the newborn rat's brain is especially immature. In human beings the sex of the brain is fixed before birth. Precisely what happens in the brain to establish its sexuality is not known, but according to a Stanford colleague of Levine, R. B. Clayton, the most likely regions where the permanent changes occur lie deep in the brain: the so-called 'medial preoptic' areas and the 'medial amygdala'.

Levine sees, in animal evolution, an ancient and profound link between sex and the brain. The method of reproduction involving two individuals, with all the business of finding, courting and mating, called for very complex patterns of behaviour, which gave advantages to the more complex brain. The way an animal behaves during reproduction is often an evocation, by chemical changes in the body, of a very elaborate pattern of activity and response which is pre-programmed in the brain.

Action and chemistry are tied together. If a male dove fails to bow and coo, because he is lacking in male hormone, a female dove in his company will not lay her eggs. Many of the 'instinctive' maternal actions of animals are evoked by hormones including, for example, the pregnant rabbit's search for nest-building materials and her plucking of hair from her own body to provide a comfortable lining for the nest. Obviously the instructions for so elaborate a performance are not contained in the hormone, which is just the key that unlocks it.

Human activities are much less stereotyped but, nevertheless, the glands and hormones interact with the brain continuously in everyday life. Nestling in the head, closely connected with the brain, is the dominant hormone-making gland of the body, the pituitary. Although formerly thought of as being its own master, the pituitary gland now looks increasingly like the agent of the brain. It provides the means whereby the brain regulates the body in a much more general way than it does through the nerves running to particular limbs and organs. The pituitary gland releases into the bloodstream a variety of hormones. The hormones are chemical messengers, travelling throughout the body, which produce very specific effects in the so-called target organs.

Although the sex hormones produced by the ovaries (in women) and the testes (in men) have the most notoriety, the other hormones are essential to life in other ways. The main glands that manufacture hormones include the thyroid in the neck, whose hormone keeps the whole body active. The adrenals, which surmount the kidneys, make their hormones in response to stress, whether of an emotional kind or due to disease and injury. But, like the sex glands, the thyroid and

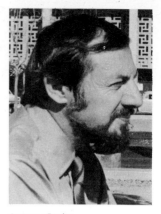

Seymour Levine.

The main hormone-producing glands of the body (below) are under the control of the pituitary (1) which is itself under the control of the brain. The other glands shown are the thyroid (2), the adrenals (3), the pancreas' 'islet cells' (4) and sex glands (5) – in the female, the ovaries.

adrenals respond to yet other hormones coming from the pituitary.

The brain and the pituitary gland are very much involved in managing the monthly cycle in women. Hormones from the pituitary stimulate the ovaries to release oestrogen, a female sex hormone. When enough oestrogen has built up in the body, the pituitary supplies a sex hormone of its own which causes the release of an egg from the ovaries. Unless the egg is fertilised during the succeeding two weeks, the woman menstruates and the cycle starts again. The brain monitors the whole process and the pineal gland (page 36) is thought to be the keeper of the calendar. The drugs used in the contraceptive pill are agents that act upon the brain, rather than the body; they deceive the brain about the state of the reproductive organs.

Vive la différence

Even without the pill, the brain responds to the influence of the changing levels of hormones circulating in the woman's blood. Part of its response is just to register the 'feedback' control of the levels of the hormones. But there are much wider responses, too. Data about women convicts tell us that a woman is four times more likely to commit a crime shortly before menstruation than at any other time. Irritability and depression at that time are, of course, commonplace, the woman's dreams are more lurid, and these effects coincide with an abrupt change in the amounts of hormones circulating in the blood. No one knows where exactly the female sex hormones 'hit' the brain, because the bloodstream carries the hormones to all parts of the brain; but there is no doubt about their impact on emotion and behaviour.

Male sex hormone also reacts upon the brain, encouraging aggressiveness, though certainly not compelling it. And there are other examples of how hormones, released on command from the brain and pituitary, return to influence the brain itself. A hormone from the pituitary promotes action aimed at self-preservation, while an excess of thyroid hormone, which activates the whole body, can also make the brain over-active and fretful.

Well-meaning people, anxious either to assert the equality of men and women or to explain homosexuality and other aberrations, have tried to minimise the inborn distinctions between the sexes. The story was that sexual attitudes and the conspicuous differences in the interests and conduct of boys and girls were acquired from the mores of family and society.   45

The proposition turns out to be essentially untrue, even though humans are much more susceptible to modification by learning than less brainy animals are. The last few years' accumulation of evidence compels us to admit that brain differences are not confined in their effects to explicit sexual acts. Transexual animals themselves show differences which are somewhat removed from sexual conduct. For example, feminised male rats go through a cycle of energetic and lazier activity, which turns out to correspond with the ovarian cycle in normal females – even though these rats have no ovaries.

Confirmation of inborn differences in males and females comes from Harry Harlow at the University of Wisconsin. He has recently been finding that, when young monkeys are separated from all adults at birth and therefore have no chance of learning how 'boys' and 'girls' ought to behave, they begin

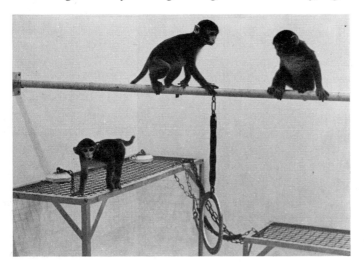

Young monkeys at play at the University of Wisconsin, after being brought up without adult company. Male and female monkeys behave differently.

to play spontaneously in the characteristic styles of their sexes. Play in young animals and humans is a serious business; as everyone now knows, it is the school for social conduct. But the bias, Harlow finds, is there from the start. Young male monkeys will wrestle and assert themselves; the females also rush about but they avoid physical contact and they never threaten the males. Baby monkeys are especially fascinating for young females, much more so than for the young males.

A reappraisal of how to secure real sexual equality among human beings may now be due. In those parts of the world where the iniquities are worst, where girls are denied a proper education and grow up to be serfs, the simple declarations of the feminists that women are the same as men is justified polemically, as a first approximation. But in countries where equality already exists in theory but not in practice, that approach has led to a dead end. Greater subtlety, taking full account of the differences built into the brains of men and women, will be required for further progress. Women are fully equal to men, intellectually, but show some tendency towards verbal skills and away from analytical skills. What is much more important, women are by nature less pushing and they are therefore less likely to succeed in a competition where men have usually written the rules. Femininity rather than feminism may have to be asserted, to secure greater esteem for the woman's way of doing things.

A repertoire of drives

The part of the brain lying by the pituitary gland is called the hypothalamus. The Swedish fluorescent techniques for making visible some of the transmitter substances in the brain can show up the activity at the point where the hypothalamus exerts direct control over the pituitary. The brain tissue normally glows green in ultraviolet light, telling of the presence of the chemical transmitter dopamine. But if the animal is pregnant, the region appears much duller. Kjell Fuxe, of the Karolinska Institute, thinks the reason why the transmitter is depleted in this case is that the brain has to work busily to prevent the pituitary from taking action inappropriate to pregnancy – namely, the release of new eggs from the ovaries.

The hypothalamus has many other functions besides the control of the pituitary gland. Lying deep inside the head, near the top of the brain stem, the hypothalamus turns out to be the region of the brain where many of our primitive drives are brought to a focus. Had its functions been known in medieval

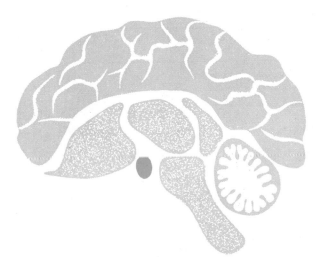

The hypothalamus, where several basic drives are organised, lies near the top of the brain stem.

times, the hypothalamus would no doubt have been designated the Devil's playground, because of its implication in gluttony, lust and the pursuit of pleasure. We can take a milder view, bearing in mind its vital importance; if we were not moved to eat we should die and without sexual desire the species would die.

Like a skilful politician, the brain is very adept at making its decisions appear to originate from somewhere else. When we feel thirsty, the impression is of a dry mouth; when we are hungry, or frightened, or over-hot, or sexually aroused, there are other characteristic feelings in the body. But all of this is misleading, because the dry mouth, stomach pangs and the rest are really the brain's own inventions. It is from the brain that the emotions and drives emanate.

Walter Hess of the University of Zurich won the Nobel prize for finding out functions of the central regions of the brain, including the hypothalamus. He it was who, between the wars, began running wires deep into the brain, in such a way as to leave the animal healthy and active but giving the experimenter the possibility of electrically stimulating regions of the brain to see what effects they produced. Stimulation with the tip of the electrode at one position in the hypothalamus would make a cat highly aggressive, so that he attacked Hess himself or any other convenient target. In contrast, stimulation at a nearby position, also in the hypothalamus, would make the cat act fearfully and try to flee. Other areas controlled digestion and excretion.

A fore-and-aft cross-section of the hypothalamus, showing the locations of particular functions. One of the regions of the brain thought to be different in men and women lies near the temperature-control site.

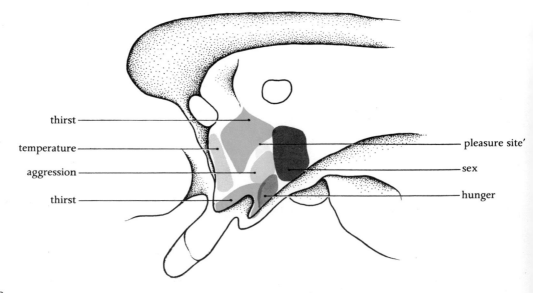

After 1950, a rapid series of discoveries about the hypothalamus, several of them at Yale University, extended and sharpened Hess's pioneering work. Eating is controlled by two kinds of sites in the hypothalamus. On either side there are 'hunger sites', where stimulation will make an animal go on eating long after he has had enough. Nearby are 'satiety sites' where stimulation will stop the hungriest animal eating. If, on the other hand, these regions are damaged, an animal will overeat and become very fat indeed.

Working normally, the hunger and satiety sites provide the necessary controls to avoid either starvation or obesity. The fact that normal humans can override their satiety sites, eating until they are bloated and still finding room for more dessert, is bad for health in an overfed society, but it gives comfort in one respect. Like the protesting hunger striker, or the thirsty men of Gideon's army who drank with decorum, the glutton gives proof that we are not completely at the mercy of these drives, deep in the brain.

The effects of hormones make it clear enough that the brain is equipped with all sorts of miniature sense organs, able to detect particular chemicals present in the blood. The hunger and satiety sites seem to operate with such detectors; in these cases, the availability of food energy in the form of glucose is what the brain is monitoring. The 'thirst sites' are interested in the salt concentration in the blood.

The brain takes care even of the apparently mundane business of keeping cool or keeping warm, using its own natural thermometers for keeping watch on the blood temperature. But when you consider how complex the body's thermostats really are, you may see why they need a brain to co-ordinate them; they involve the control of the blood vessels of the skin, the kidneys and the thyroid, of breathing rate and shivering, of feelings of hunger and thirst, and other mechanisms, too. The main 'temperature sites' in the brain seem to be in the so-called 'pre-optic' regions of the hypothalamus.

In 1953 José Delgado, Warren Roberts and Neal Miller, at Yale, showed that stimulation of particular areas of the brain stem was evidently unpleasant for the animal – he acted as if frightened or in pain. It was by an accident that the next very interesting feature of the hypothalamus was discovered. In the same year, working in Donald Hebb's group in Canada, James Olds was looking to see whether stimulation of the brain stem of a rat could cause reactions of apparent pleasure in the animal. Olds hit upon what he was looking for – but only by a very clumsy aim which put the tip of the electrode higher in the brain than he intended.

Working with Peter Milner, Olds found that the areas of the brain where stimulation gave the greatest pleasure were spread through the hypothalamus from front to back – a 'river of reward'. In the McGill experiments, the rats were tested by allowing them to switch on the current to the electrode by pressing a treadle. Some rats pressed the treadle every two seconds for 24 hours without stopping and a hungry rat would often pass up a chance to eat, preferring to stimulate his 'pleasure site'.

The hypothalamus also contains 'aversion sites', where an animal responds to stimulation as if frightened or in pain. But at some locations the resulting actions of the animal are very mixed up indeed: the stimulation seems both pleasurable and disagreeable to the animal. In one experiment at Yale, a rat with an electrode in such a location had the opportunity to switch on the stimulation by pressing a treadle and then switch it off again by turning a wheel. And the animal did exactly that, over and over again, rushing from the wheel to the treadle and back again.

And an electrode in a 'sex site' towards the back of the hypothalamus, on either side, will provoke sexual excitement, up to orgasm, in a rat. If the animal is able to stimulate himself he may go on doing so until he collapses with exhaustion. 'Killing sites' occur on the two sides of the hypothalamus of wild rats. Pierre Karli of the University of Strasbourg reported their discovery in 1956; if they are removed, a rat that normally kills any mouse put into his cage will no longer do so.

The finding of 'pleasure sites', where stimulation produced no particular action but only evident gratification, prompted some speculation that animals and men were indeed pure hedonists at heart, striving only for the excitement of these regions of the hypothalamus. Provocative though the discovery is, no such conclusion is yet warranted. The pleasure sites appear to be associated particularly with feeding and sex and plainly only a small part of our lives is spent in direct enjoyment of these pleasures.

In any case, the effect of direct intervention in the hypothalamus, of an automaton-like response, is no more representative of normal conduct than the fact that electrical stimulation elsewhere in the brain will make an animal (or a man) raise a limb involuntarily. The drives like hunger and sex are very necessary for survival, but they are only a part of a more complex system, involving emotions like fear, anger and love, which in turn are only components of the even more complex

systems of the whole brain and the whole individual.

A group of cages at the University of Wisconsin made up a monkey equivalent of the human suburbia. Each cage contained a family unit of father, mother and children – the so-called nuclear family. Although conventional by human standards, it was not at all normal for the adult male rhesus monkey, who leads a promiscuous life and is not particularly attached to the mother or her children; certainly he is not usually confined with the baby. In this arrangement of cages, the youngsters could go out in the 'street' connecting all the cages, and visit one another's home, but the adults were forced to stay with their mates by the simple device of making the front door too small for them.

This experiment to see how monkeys would react to domestic life on human lines was well under way in 1970. It was set up by Margaret Harlow, wife and collaborator of Harry Harlow, as the latest of their studies of the tender emotions of family love. On a visit to this little monkey community at siesta time, one could glimpse the relationships at work. As one family crowded together on a narrow shelf for a rest, the youngest squeezed between his father and mother; the father, having had enough of this, found a ledge of his own on which to rest. One of the neighbour's daughters, fascinated by the baby, was in visiting, overstaying her welcome and making a nuisance of herself.

Mrs Harlow told of her surprise at how well the monkeys had adapted to this unnatural life with father. Evidently the human family is not a ridiculous or unworkable convention, even among these distant primate relatives. The fathers played with the young monkeys, especially the males, more than males usually do; they were quite rough with them, but the youngsters evidently enjoyed it and kept coming back for more. As a result, they were much bolder with the human experimenters. 'They are the most self-confident, self-sufficient and courageous young monkeys we've ever seen', Mrs Harlow remarked.

Her most serious interest was in the process whereby the young monkey switched from clinging to mother to leading an almost independent life with monkeys of his own age what in humans we call cutting the apron strings. It is an essential process in the maturing of the young monkey and the mother begins to repulse him, gently but firmly, with increasing frequency. Yet it is a slow business and is not complete even by two years of age.

'We are happy to state that we now believe that. . . real mothering is here to stay!' Harry and Margaret Harlow thus testified in 1966, after many years already spent experimenting with baby monkeys at the University of Wisconsin. Although the Harlows have been careful to point out that monkey research cannot give total understanding of human beings, the parallels with human family love are very plausible. Of their classic studies of the nature of love, Harry Kay of Sheffield has predicted that it will be seen as a milestone, as more psychologists turn their attention to human virtues as well as vices. What is more virtuous than a mother's loving kindness towards her children?

In this age of incessant psychological advice, many human parents are rather calculating in bringing up their children.

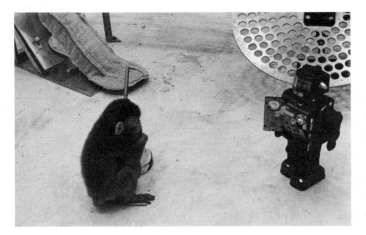

The young monkey is clinging to the cloth-covered stand, which he regards as his mother, because he is frightened of the toy robot.

Young monkeys separated from their mothers at birth often adopt the characteristic 'choo-choo' formation (right) for mutual comfort.

The monkey mother is an innocent caricature of the human mother. For the first three or four months of the monkey baby's life (perhaps matching the first eighteen months for a human baby) the mother is all comfort and protection. During this first stage, as the Harlows put it, the baby can do no wrong. There is almost no punishment, and the mother watches the baby anxiously when he first crawls beyond her arm's reach. There follows a transitional stage, in which the mother gradually begins to discipline the baby and sometimes to reject him, while still protecting him. Finally, in many species of monkeys, the birth of a new baby makes the mother quite suddenly and completely reject the older one. An adult male often comes along to cherish the youngster and so relieve the anxiety of separation from the mother.

Meanwhile the young monkey has been passing through several stages in learning to love his mother and also other young monkeys. When newborn, his clinging to mother is a

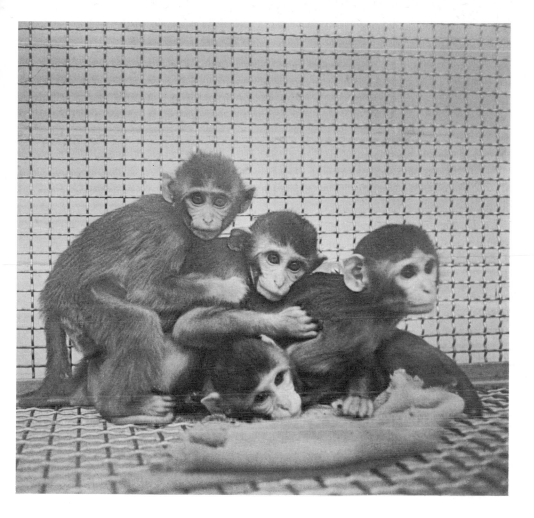

merc reflex; only after two or three weeks is he doing so voluntarily, so that a true relationship can be established with the mother – the 'comfort and attachment stage', in the Harlows' terminology. By his third month, the monkey is learning by imitating his mother. There follows a stage in which the mere presence of the mother becomes sufficient to give the young monkey a feeling of security as he explores the world around. He also begins to play with other young monkeys and the additional affection so formed gradually becomes more important than the ties to the mother.

Harry Harlow broke severely into this natural pattern, in his experiments with baby monkeys. He separated them from their mothers. To some he gave human mothers; to others he gave imitation mothers, dolls covered with cloth; to others again he gave more 'brutal' imitation mothers, wire frames of the right sort of shape and size but uncomforting to the touch. He prevented or forced the contacts between infant monkeys of the same age. By altering all aspects of the young monkey's experience, in a controlled fashion, he sought to discover what part 'learning to love' plays in the life of the monkey.

Here are some of the conclusions. Bodily contact is so much sought after by the young monkey that he will cling to a doll, or to another young monkey, if there is no other mother to be had. A young monkey raised with a cloth mother learns to rely on it for security and may be terrified if it is absent, though the sense of security is less valuable than that given by monkey or human mothers. The monkey's love for its cloth mother will persist for years. No comparable affection develops for a bare wire mother, even if it is the young monkey's source of food.

Too little mothering (cloth mother) or too much mothering (confinement with the mother) impairs the ability of a monkey to learn to play with other monkeys of the same age. A monkey raised in complete isolation for its first six months suffers social devastation. When released among other monkeys of the same age he is quite unable to play with them; nor does he learn to do so after many weeks of exposure to normal social contacts but shows aggressive tendencies towards adult or even baby monkeys. If a female so treated in infancy should herself become pregnant, she will reject her own baby. But recently Harry Harlow and Stephen Soumi have found that a playful younger monkey can act as 'therapist' for a deprived monkey.

One more of the Harlows' conclusions deserves special note because of its relevance to perennially-disputed questions about the influences of upbringing on the intellectual capacity of children. I should say possible relevance, because in intellect a human child differs greatly from a monkey, so that comparisons are uncertain. Nevertheless, the Harlows reported that, however deprived a young monkey was, socially, and whatever the emotional cost of that upbringing, there was no detectable difference in the monkey's ability to solve problems, after training had overcome the emotional barriers to participation in tests.

The organisation of emotion

Uwe Jurgens pressed a switch and a squirrel monkey sitting in his laboratory let out a call. Electrical stimulation of the monkey's brain produced this call at will. Among the monkeys and apes, the squirrel monkey has the largest known repertoire of cackles, peeps, shrieks and other calls. Jurgens was engaged in mapping the areas of the brain involved in different kinds of calls. Afterwards, the monkey would go into a cage with the choice of having the brain stimulation and not having it, depending on his position in the cage. In this way, the monkey

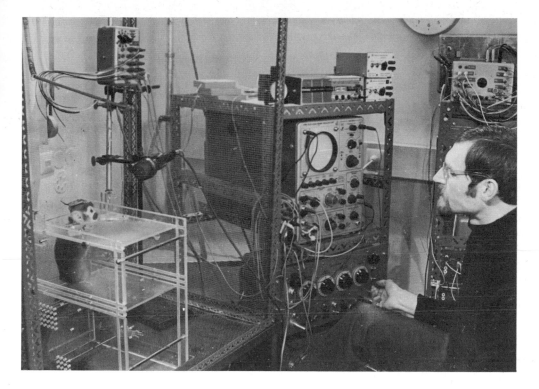

This squirrel monkey produces a particular call in response to electrical stimulation of a particular part of the brain, in an experiment by Uwe Jurgens.

himself would show whether the call was associated with an agreeable or an unpleasant emotion, by deciding where to sit.

'Monkey talk' is simply a means whereby one animal lets his companions know his emotional state. Up till now, observers of animal behaviour have not yet been able to tell exactly how an animal is feeling. At the Max-Planck Institute of Psychiatry in Munich, where Jurgens works, prolonged studies of the calls and gestures used by the squirrel monkeys in their social life have helped to open the way to finding out, in detail, how the brain produces different kinds of emotion. At the same time, the effects that each call or gesture have on the other monkeys are important for understanding the social interactions of the monkeys. Detlev Ploog, who leads this research in Munich, explains the motives:

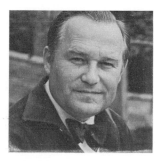

Detlev Ploog: 'The single monkey is only half a monkey'.

The single monkey is only half a monkey. Its normal life is shaped by interactions with its companions. In human life, communication with one another is the main factor. As a psychiatrist, I believe that the cause of mental illness is a disturbance or even a breakdown of the communication system. But the human communication system is very elaborate and we cannot experiment with patients. That's why, at a psychiatric institute, we investigate the gestures and calls of these animals.

55

Monkeys under remote control may seem like a story out of science fiction, but they figure routinely in research at the Munich institute, as in some American laboratories. For years the way monkeys behave in groups has been carefully watched and analysed, both in the wild and in big communal cages. By gestures and calls the monkeys organise their social life, establishing who is the dominant male, who the favourite female and so on. But now, implant a bunch of electrodes in the brain and leave them in place in a squirrel monkey living in the communal cage, and you have the means of producing an unexpected, uncharacteristic gesture by the monkey any time you like.

Manfred Maurus runs such experiments in Ploog's group. To a little receiver mounted in a cap on the monkey's head he can transmit a signal which will then stimulate a preselected region of the monkey's brain. In response, a non-dominant male can act quite out of character, challenging the dominant male by a genital display or some other chosen gesture, or by open attack. The reactions of the other monkeys can then be recorded, sharpening the understanding of natural communications in the group. Now the 'telestimulation' technique is being extended to the vocal calls as well. It is as if an experimenter from another planet, seeking the nuances of meaning of the human wolf-whistle, made a clergyman suddenly give it, and watched the reactions of the bystanders.

Gestures and other signals, comparable with those in monkeys, play a part in human life, too. In spite of the great overlay of language in our dealings with one another, non-verbal

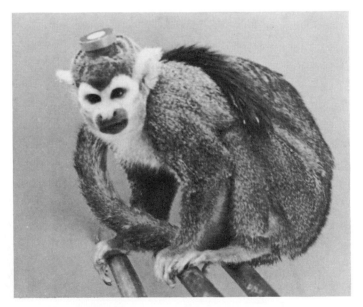

A squirrel monkey wearing the receiver cap connected to deep regions of his brain. He will respond in predictable ways to signals transmitted to a chosen point. This subordinate male will attack the 'boss' monkey in obedience to a stimulus.

signals, often registered quite unconsciously, remain particularly important for indicating the emotional state and social attitude of the moment. In the last few years psychologists have begun to take more interest in them. Facial expressions, with different kinds of smiles and frowns, are obvious enough; so are laughter and tears, the blanched face of fear and the red face of embarrassment. But some are subtler, including the direction of our glances when talking, and how closely we approach another person. National differences in non-verbal signalling are a frequent source of misunderstanding, like the placating grin of the Chinese who has offended.

Biologists accustomed to studying animal signals have been looking with a fresh eye at the unsophisticated gestures of children around the age of four. A group at Birmingham University led by Michael Chance has found, for example, that when a child raises his hand as if to strike, the position of the hand in relation to the head is a quite exact indicator of how aggressive or defensive he feels. Other children can read the signals perfectly well and react accordingly. Remnants of these gestures are commonplace in adults; stroking the back of one's neck is a sign of defensiveness, adapted from the child's most defensive 'beating posture'.

Changes in the size of the pupils of the eyes are an unconscious form of communication: large pupils denote interest and therefore make a woman seem more attractive. (Modified detail from Botticelli's Primavera*)*

The size of the pupils of the eyes is another giveaway. In 1960 Eckhard Hess of the University of Chicago noticed that he needed less light to read by when he was especially interested in the book. His excitement made his pupils bigger, thereby admitting more light. In subsequent tests he found, for example, that a woman's pupils would grow big seeing the

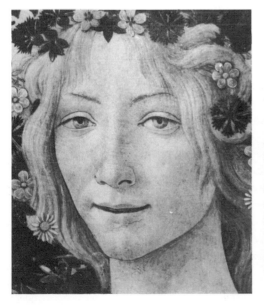
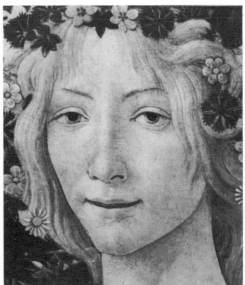

picture of a baby and a man's would enlarge for a nude woman. Cold dislike would produce a narrowing. The response to a corpse and other shocking sights is enlargement followed by shrinkage. During a mental task, such as working out an anagram, the pupils become gradually bigger and return to normal when the problem is solved.

Dozens of institutes now record pupil changes for purposes ranging from psychiatric diagnosis to evaluating tv commercials. But long before present-day psychologists took up the subject, women were using belladonna to enlarge their pupils to make themselves more attractive, while some salesmen and poker players knew how to detect the signs of pleasure in another man's pupils.

Our emotional responses are organised chiefly in a federation of regions in and around the top of the brain stem, known as the limbic system. In a monkey the arrangement is similar. What Detlev Ploog finds particularly fascinating is that the same system is heavily involved in determining how a monkey will behave socially and what gestures and calls he will make. Emotions are not feelings supplied gratuitously by nature; they serve very practical purposes, for aiding appropriate reactions to events and to other individuals, and for eliciting responses from others.

The hypothalamus, lying at the core of the limbic system, exerts its influence on the internal state of the body as a whole. It does so through the pituitary gland and also through an elaborate network of nerves which controls the rate of breathing, the width of the blood vessels, the heart-rate and so on. These bodily circumstances react upon the brain as a whole so that high blood pressure, for example, can reinforce feelings of agitation. But this system is not operating in isolation: it is directly coupled with many other parts of the brain and indirectly with them all. Although the hypothalamus seems to be particularly concerned with the primitive drives of hunger, thirst and sex, more elaborate emotional organisation occurs in adjacent central regions in the brain, where feelings of anger, fear and ecstasy are generated.

Certain parts of the roof of the brain are also involved in emotional organisation, especially the temporal lobes on either side of the head, and evidently also the great frontal lobes, the activities of which have been somewhat mysterious for investigators. José Delgado tells of patients made very flirtatious during brain operations by electrical stimulation below the surface of the temporal lobes. 'I'd like to be a girl', said one boy with homosexual tendencies.

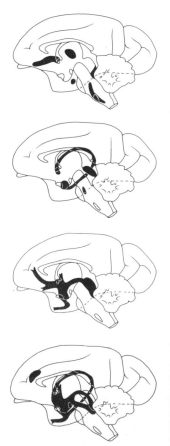

Maps of the regions of the squirrel monkey's brain involved in various kinds of calls indicate the organisation of the particular emotions associated with each call. Large areas deep in the brain are involved in emotional states. In descending order, the calls are 'chirping', which is a means of attracting attention, 'shrieking' (high excitement), 'cackling' (general aggressiveness), 'growling' (aggressiveness directed at a particular animal). (After Jurgens)

Other brain connections, not yet fully traced, allow the emotions to bias our perceptions of reality. The intensity of a pain depends upon the sufferer's state of mind. Twenty years ago Jerome Bruner found that poor children and well-off children did not see coins in the same way; the poor children judged the coins to be physically larger than they really were. In more recent experiments at the Applied Psychology Research Unit in Cambridge, Donald Broadbent and Margaret Gregory have found that emotionally-loaded words such as 'death' and 'blood' are harder to hear correctly than are neutral words like 'square' and 'run', when there is confusion by a background noise.

Emotional states can also, of course, produce physical damage in the body. A famous report of 1958 from the US Army Medical Department told of stomach and duodenal ulcers caused in executive monkeys. Two monkeys sat side

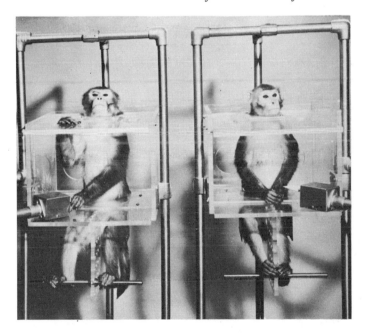

The 'executive monkey' experiment. The animal at the left had to press his lever to avoid shocks to both animals, and tended to suffer gastric ulcers while the 'passenger' did not.

by side. One of them was the executive; whenever a red light was showing he had to press a lever at least once every twenty seconds, otherwise both monkeys received an electric shock. After about three weeks, the executive monkey succumbed to a duodenal ulcer; his companion, who received just as many shocks but had no responsibility, was unaffected.

Closer studies showed that the excess stomach acid giving rise to the ulcers was produced, not during the working sessions, but when the red light was out. Moreover, only a routine six hours' work followed by six hours off caused actual ulcers; no other schedule, even the most strenuous, was effective. It made a nice story, fitting in with popular ideas about the hard-working, ulcer-prone human executive; but experiments with executive rats, done ten years later at Yale University, have contradicted it.

The executive rat had to press a switch, whenever a light came on and the floor shook, to save himself and his companion from an electric shock. In experiments of this kind, Jay

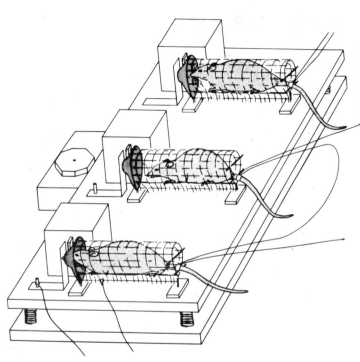

The 'executive rat' experiments. One animal had to press a switch with his nose to avoid the shock. This study gave results opposite to those of the 'executive monkey' experiment.

Weiss found that the non-executive 'yoked' animal was more likely to suffer the severe stomach ulcers. A possible explanation for the opposite results of the US Army group is that the executive monkeys were chosen because of their aptitude in working the lever – thereby introducing a temperamental bias from the outset. Whatever the reason, Weiss is confident that, in animals in general, the opportunity to cope with a stress reduces, rather than increases, its effects.

The most emotional animal

The foregoing pages have made a great deal out of animal experimentation. How relevant is it to our own lives and brains? Are not human beings much more the masters of their emotions than the lower animals?

The citizens of a modern city, going about their business efficiently and politely, seem less prone to emotional disturbances than a pack of wolves or a gang of monkeys. But Donald Hebb believes that appearances are very misleading in this respect, as he explains in the remarks overleaf (page 63). He has important theoretical reasons for his view of man as the most emotional of animals. Earlier (page 34) Hebb's general description of arousal and emotion was given; up to a certain point, arousal produces heightened alertness and interest, which then gives way to emotional disturbance and anxiety. The more complex the brain, the more vulnerable it is to emotional disturbance.

But Hebb also believes that man's intellect and emotional characteristics give him a greater aptitude for altruism than any other animal. Dogs, dolphins and chimpanzees are known to form durable friendships of one individual with another. Friendship may give no obvious advantage to a selfish animal and indeed it can involve the animal in exerting or endangering itself to help its friend. Altruism is not necessarily asssociated with happy emotions. A chimpanzee cannot avoid sharing his food with a hungry companion who begs for it, any more than a human mother can ignore for long the cries of her baby, but they may both respond very bad-temperedly.

Altruism plainly gives advantages to animals living in groups. There is no reason to suppose that man is deficient compared with the other animals in this respect. On the contrary, our brains are very well supplied with machinery for altruism and the more tender emotions. Our high foreheads are perhaps an outward sign of the special provision at the front of the brain for sensitivity in our human relationships, while our powers of language, housed in the left side of the brain, increase their precision. Our acute faculties of self-awareness and self-criticism are also part of the same story, and so is our peculiar pattern, or lack of pattern, in sexual activity. The fact that human sexuality is not seasonal, except to a very slight degree, contrasts with the usual on-off pattern in animals. It helps in the cementing of human relationships and in making possible the more tender aspects of sexual love.

Sir Wilfred Le Gros Clark of Oxford University observed a few years ago:

> It now seems pretty certain that it was the development of the distinctively human type of social organisation, depending in the first instance on the use of tools and weapons in co-operative activities for foraging and hunting for food and for the protection of family groups, which demanded an ac-

celerated development of those parts of the brain whereby emotional and instinctive impulses can be more effectively subordinated to the good of the community as a whole.

We have seen some striking examples of the coupling between the brain and the rest of the body. Other very recent and exciting discoveries have transformed our estimation of this interaction, especially of the influence of mental processes on the glands and organs of the body. The transformation merits a chapter to itself (Chapter 5). Before that we turn to some of the ways in which knowledge of brain mechanisms can be applied to control of the human mind.

Donald Hebb (right) and his opinion on human emotionality. The childish tantrum (below) is mild compared with the intensity of emotion which human adults can generate and therefore try to avoid (below, right).

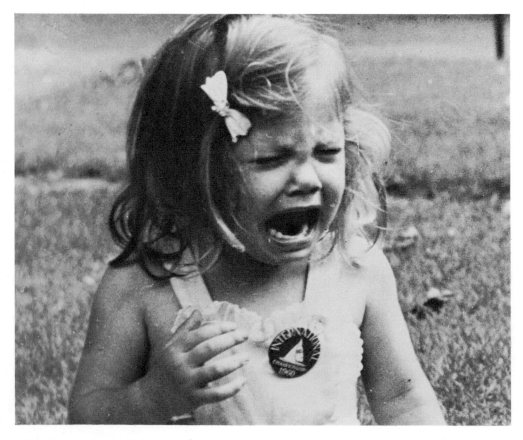

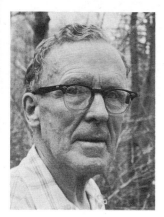

Man is probably the most emotional animal of all. Nobody would seriously suggest for a moment that the spider is capable of emotional disturbance. The rat may be capable of some fear but that's about all. In the dog we have something more complex. The dog is capable of jealousy, of grief for a missing master and certainly of fear. But with the chimpanzee we get something that's very human. The chimpanzee that is teased in feeding may sulk for weeks; shown a death-mask he may be utterly panic-stricken.

Notice that progression – as the brain becomes more complex with evolution, as we become more intelligent, we become more vulnerable to emotion. The human child with his temper tantrums provides us with the clearest example of pure, unadulterated emotion. He grows out of it we say. If he does I'm wrong. My theory says that the human adult is more emotional than the three-year-old.

Why don't we seem that way? Well, how often has a neighbour spoken insultingly to you? How often have you had to handle a corpse? How often have you heard laughter at a funeral? We build human society so that we are carefully protected from our own emotional weaknesses, because we are so easily upset.

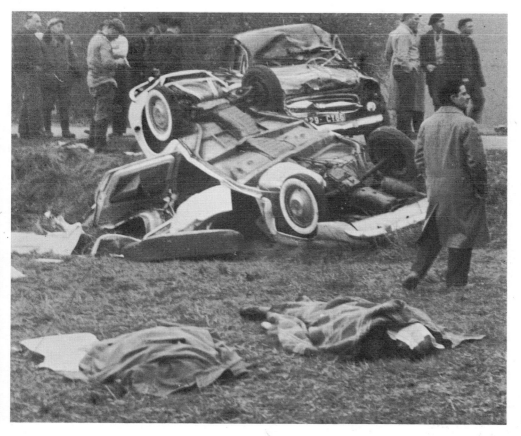

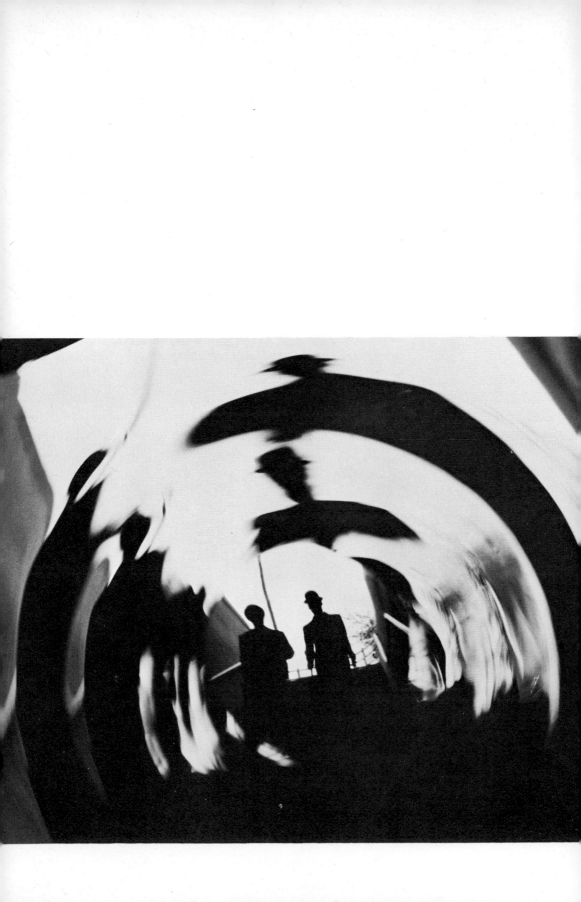

4 Control of the Mind

A weak electric current delivered to a chosen part of the brain can control specific activity, while a drug in the bloodstream can distort or improve general mental processes. Fears about political abuses of mind-controlling techniques are not unfounded, but human individuality provides some defences.

At Alamogordo in New Mexico, in 1969, a little artificial island was occupied by a chimpanzee. A nearby computer was in two-way radio communication with the animal's brain, bringing it to a limited extent under computer control. Wires ran into the brain. From two of them the radio transmitted, to the computer, information about electric activity in a particular region, the 'almond' or amygdala, deep in the side of the brain. Another pair of wires ran into the stem of the brain, to points where stimulation was evidently unpleasant to the chimpanzee. At any rate, it acted as a deterrent.

The computer was set to detect a particular electric pattern in the brain which was a mark of boisterousness. Whenever it did so, it worked the punishing electrodes in the brain stem, again by radio. That pattern was almost completely suppressed after a number of sessions with the computer turned on. The overall effect was to change a lively, rather aggressive chimpanzee into a very quiet and docile animal. When the computer

Remote control of an animal's brain by computer. A pair of wires registers events deep in the chimpanzee's brain; another pair punishes a certain type of electric activity, detected by the computer.

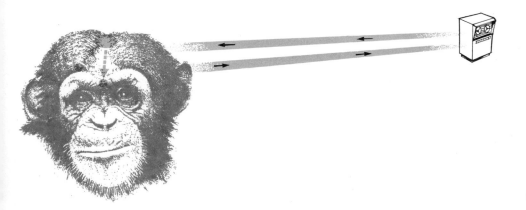

was switched off the animal returned to normal after about two weeks. This experiment was run at the Holloman Air Force Base by experimenters from Yale University.

Also at Alamogordo, just a quarter of a century ago in the test known as Trinity, the first A-bomb explosion occurred and changed the world. For anyone impressed by the potential uses of electrodes (wires implanted in the human brain) for good or evil, this geographical coincidence of fateful experiments may seem noteworthy. But just how significant, for the human future, is the ever-growing range of possibilities for direct control of the mind, by this and other techniques?

Electrodes in the brain already have serious purposes, for research and for treatment of the sick. They have helped in identifying the functions of deep-lying regions of the brain and

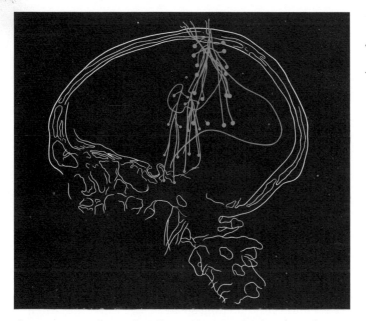

Electrodes implanted in a human brain. The paths followed by the fine gold wires are diagrammed from an X-ray photograph. The patient is a young epileptic.

they assist in the study of emotion in animals. Many human beings lead a normal life with wires in their heads left over from brain operations. In a typical case the surgeon stimulates the brain to discover the site of a disorder and then uses the same electrodes to destroy the offending brain tissue with an electric current. Less harm is done by leaving the wires in place than by removing them.

A much smaller number of humans are wired for more or less continuous stimulation of their brains. In London, Giles Brindley is trying to help blind people to see, by implanting an array of wires into the area at the back of the brain which normally receives signals from the eyes. The first operation of this kind enabled the patient to report spots of light when the electrodes were activated. Brindley's second attempt was in preparation in the summer of 1970. Given large numbers of electrodes connected to suitable photo-electrical devices, Brindley expects that blind people will be able to recognise visual patterns, and eventually to read print.

Elsewhere, surgeons have laid active wires to more private regions of the human brain. New Orleans has some fame, or notoriety, as a place where human beings go around with active electrodes in their heads. There, Robert Heath of Tulane University has reported on patients who are free to stimulate their own brains, by pressing buttons that send impulses to wires terminating in various regions. The patient will find the button that makes him feel good, and go on pressing it many times over. One much-fancied place for electric self-stimulation is the so-called septal region, deep in the front of the brain, where the electric stimulus produces sexual feelings. Procedures of this kind, used in humans, have come in for strenuous criticism on ethical grounds and the possible damage to the brain is not negligible.

José Delgado, a Spanish-born medical scientist at Yale, is another who has made many studies with electrodes in the brains of animals and humans. His team was responsible for chimpanzee pacification by computer, as at Alamogordo. For humans, he looks forward to the day when computers will be linked by radio to human brains, here to suppress an incipient epileptic fit, there to prevent a homicidal outburst in a mental patient.

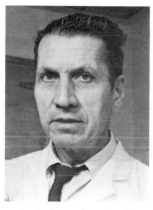

José Delgado. As the author of diverse experiments in the physical control of brain processes, Delgado talks of a turning-point in evolution, 'at which the mind can be used to influence its own structure, functions and purposes'.

Once when he was visiting his homeland, Delgado staged a mock bullfight. Photographs of the event were widely published and showed a charging bull that skidded to a halt whenever a radio signal stimulated his brain. With his book on *Physical Control of the Mind* (1968), Delgado has established himself as the chief prophet of a better world built with brain electrodes. He is at pains to emphasise the limitations of electrical stimulation of the brain, but he sees it as an invaluable tool for helping the mentally sick to recover and the criminally minded to reform.

His proposals raise an interesting legal and philosophical conundrum. If a man commits a crime while he has active electrodes in his brain, who is to blame – himself or his doctor? More generally, Delgado's hopes are other people's fears. For them, Big Brother appears with a new technology for political control. So far, it is very hard to imagine the logistics whereby a dictator could arrange all the surgery needed to put precisely positioned wires into the heads of all his citizens, against their will.

Classes of people who might be particularly accessible to implants of this kind include convicts, prisoners of war and patients in hospital. Otherwise the greatest source of danger in mind control by this method may be in members of the public volunteering for brain implants. They could do it 'for kicks' already, on the basis of existing technology. Wires giving a strong feeling of pleasure might create a kind of electrical addiction. More serious citizens may in due course come to want electrodes for other purposes, such as achieving direct communication with computers or with one another. At present, no one really knows how to begin wiring brains for such purposes.

How mind drugs work

In any case, why speculate about the wholesale use of implanted electrodes, when other, very powerful techniques are already commonplace for direct intervention in the workings of the mind – namely, with drugs? Advances in brain research have helped to explain how known drugs influence mood or create delusions, and other potent drugs may now be invented less accidentally than hitherto. Meanwhile, some of the new mind drugs have transformed the lives of many mentally ill people. They have also given scientists a valuable aid in investigations of the natural chemistry of the brain. At the same time, their freelance use by pill fanciers and acidheads has raised hot issues in what Timothy Leary calls 'the politics of ecstasy' but others label less euphorically.

The natural drugs, the plant extracts and fermentations with which men have comforted or blown their minds since prehistoric times, anticipated several man-made types of greater purity and potency. Modern chemistry knows the active principles in the traditional materials, for instance the tranquilliser reserpine in the *Rauwolfia* root of traditional Indian medicine, and the maddening agent psilocin in 'God's flesh', the Mexican sacred mushroom. LSD was foreshadowed in the grimmest way by the St Anthony's Fire (or 'dancing mania') of medieval times, the painful and fatal madness of poisoning by ergot, a fungus that grows on damp rye. The LSD-25, which first astonished the Swiss chemist Albert Hofmann with its mental effects in 1943, was derived from ergot.

LSD is the sacred acid of the present-day psychedelic cult and even the technical jargon becomes polemical. 'Psychedelic' means mind-expanding. The alternative name for drugs of this class, 'psychotomimetic', means psychosis-imitating or, more simply, maddening. The madness is only temporary in most

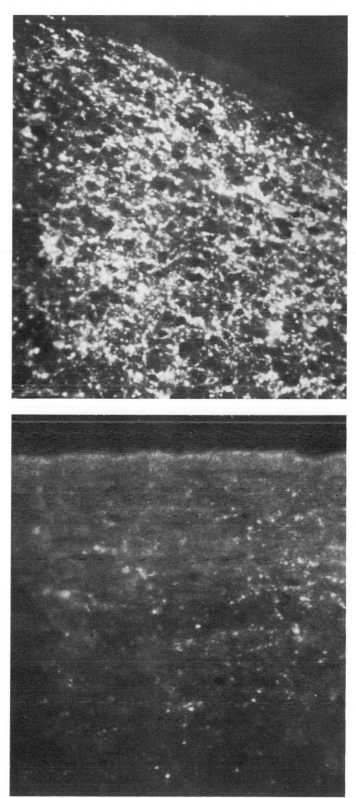

Drug action made visible. The upper photograph shows brain cells under the microscope, with a natural chemical transmitter (noradrenalin) shown up brightly by the Swedish fluorescence technique. In the lower photograph, the same area of the brain is seen after treatment with reserpine, a tranquillising drug, which reduces the amount of noradrenalin available.
(Microphotographs by K. Fuxe)

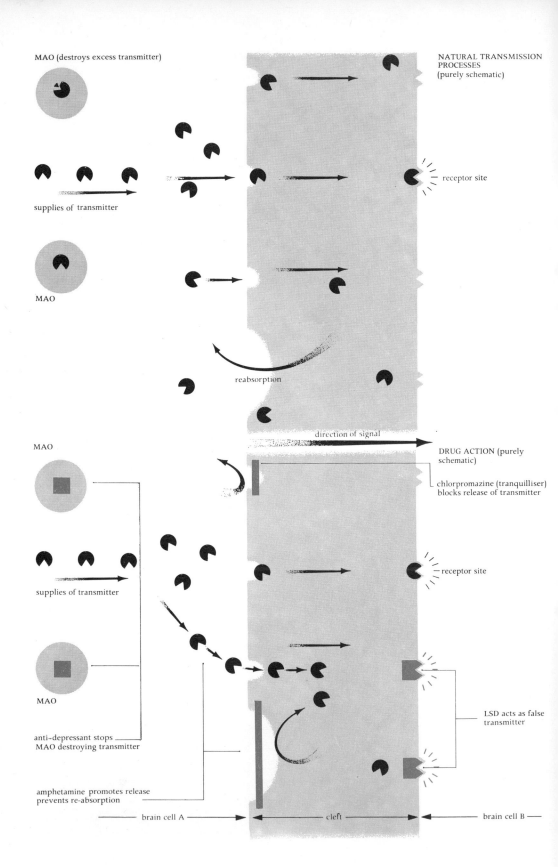

MAO (destroys excess transmitter)

NATURAL TRANSMISSION PROCESSES
(purely schematic)

receptor site

supplies of transmitter

MAO

reabsorption

direction of signal

DRUG ACTION (purely schematic)

chlorpromazine (tranquilliser) blocks release of transmitter

MAO

supplies of transmitter

receptor site

MAO

LSD acts as false transmitter

anti-depressant stops MAO destroying transmitter

amphetamine promotes release prevents re-absorption

brain cell A ——— | ——— cleft ——— | ——— brain cell B ———

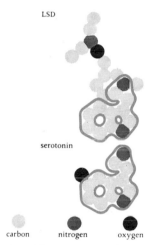

LSD

serotonin

carbon   nitrogen   oxygen

The maddening properties of LSD are thought to be due to its similarity, in part of its chemical structure, to the natural brain chemical, serotonin.

cases and the distortions of perception, the illusions, the feelings of insight, ecstasy and anguish produced by such drugs have often been described. The claim by the cult that LSD is also an aphrodisiac, sexually exciting, is classical propaganda that need not be taken seriously. The value of the LSD 'trip' in psychiatry is a matter of continuing controversy.

The only grounds for hesitation in applying the term 'maddening' to drugs of the LSD type is that other drugs can also produce insane experience and conduct. Julius Axelrod, of the National Institutes of Health in Maryland, is a leading authority on the mind drugs; he takes the view that the classical madness of paranoid schizophrenia is better mimicked by the effects of amphetamine rather than LSD. Amphetamine is usually classified as a stimulant, in distinction from the psychotomimetic (or psychedelic) drugs.

Like some other psychotomimetic drugs (including the psilocin of the Mexican mushroom), LSD is chemically very similar to serotonin, a material occurring naturally in the brain. Serotonin is one of the transmitters that carry messages across the narrow gaps between certain brain cells. LSD takes effect by jamming the natural transmitter system. Opinions differ as to what exactly happens but one view is that the LSD arrives as a pseudo-transmitter and over-activates many brain cells. The brain seems to try unsuccessfully to protect itself by bottling up the natural transmitter. The quantities of natural transmitter in the brain are really very small, so that very small amounts of LSD make a big difference. Mescaline is a drug producing similar mental effects, but chemically it resembles another natural transmitter in the brain, noradrenalin.

The ways in which other classes of mind drugs operate can be told more precisely. They, too, interfere with the chemical transmissions from brain cell to brain cell. Common sense suggests that the tranquillisers should reduce the level of brain activity and, for once in a while, common sense is correct. One of them, reserpine, reduces the amount of noradrenalin in the brain cells while another, chlorpromazine, blocks its release. Either way, fewer messages pass between those brain cells that use noradrenalin as their transmitter and the information from the senses is less demanding. The tranquillisers are valuable drugs for psychiatrists, in controlling the symptoms of schizophrenia and of anxiety states in general.

The best-known stimulant or 'pep' drug, amphetamine, has the opposite effect. It increases the amount of noradrenalin active between brain cells. Amphetamine encourages the release of the transmitter from storage in the cells and it tends to prevent the process whereby noradrenalin is normally re-   71 absorbed by the cells. The drug may also act directly on those 'receptor' regions of the target cells which respond to the natural transmitter. Amphetamine makes some people feel very elated but its general effect is mental over-excitement, with wakefulness, 'edginess' and a racing pulse.

In principle, stimulants like amphetamine can help to relieve depression due to weak transmission between brain cells, but a newer class of drugs is preferred for this purpose – the anti-depressants. These are slower but surer in their results. Some of them, including iproniazid, block the natural agents (enzymes) which restrict the amount of chemical transmitters available in the brain. These anti-depressants are called MAO-inhibitors but have nothing to do with counter-revolution in China. The MAOs in question are the mono-amine oxidases, enzymes which normally destroy excess transmitter sub-stances in the brain. As MAOs also cope with materials present in food, particularly in cheese, patients on anti-depressants have to be careful about what they eat.

Such are the main categories of mind drugs available for the treatment of the mentally sick. Other important agents, includ-ing the lithium salts that relieve mania, do not fit in this list, but to prolong it would be tedious. These mind drugs must be rated quite differently, in potency and effect, from traditional milder drugs – tea, coffee, tobacco, alcohol and so on – all of which are admittedly dangerous in excess. As we shall see, there are other kinds of mind drugs producing effects that psychiatrists are unlikely ever to want, but which imply pos-sible methods of mind control for more sinister purposes.

Tyrant's pharmacy?

Military planners have not overlooked mind drugs as potential weapons. The nerve gases, among the deadliest of existing chemical weapons, attack the nerves of the body rather than the mind but, like the psychiatric drugs, they intervene in the natural transmission of signals between nerve cells. American chemical munitions are known to include an 'incapacitating agent', BZ, the declared toxic symptoms of which include mental slowness, dizziness, disorientation, hallucinations and sometimes maniacal outbursts. Its composition is secret and independent commentators give conflicting suggestions about what BZ may be. It does not sound quite like LSD and may well be a mild 'nerve gas' acting primarily on the nerves of the body.

LSD and similar drugs could probably be spread effectively over enemy troops; the doses required are very small. Not many years ago, films showing a cat cowering from a mouse and soldiers throwing their guns away, after treatment with LSD, encouraged fanciful talk of war without death. But the snags are fairly obvious: the result of general madness in the enemy in a battle situation is very hard to predict, and the overdoses inevitable in many cases would cause permanent insanity or death. In practice, whatever specific purpose the non-lethal gas is supposed to serve, there are usually agents of more precision and predictability than LSD.

All sorts of special mental effects have been claimed for drugs; many more have figured in science fiction and thrillers. At a time when brain and drug research are advancing faster than ever before, it is not always easy to tell fact from fancy in the tales of chemicals that might control the human mind. Here are some examples.

Truth drugs. The truth is that these materials (sodium amytal for example) scarcely work in the way they are sometimes alleged to do, in making a prisoner give up lying or tell facts that he would not otherwise divulge. They are basically just anaesthetics that make a person drowsy. What he tells then is no more likely to be the truth than what he would say if he were drunk.

Memory drugs. Almost any of us might wish for a better memory and the ability to learn faster. For more than half a century it has been known that a small dose of strychnine accelerates learning in rats. During the past ten years the possibility has emerged of giving strychnine or other materials, even after learning, to enhance the memory. But there have been no systematic studies in humans. Trials of the drug known as magnesium pemoline, said to promote memory in old people, were inconclusive. There are also claims that knowledge itself can actually be injected in chemical form (see page 118).

Amnesia drugs. These, too, anticipate a later chapter, where we shall find certain antibiotics wiping out memory in goldfish and other animals (see page 122). These drugs prevent information passing from a short-term memory store into the long-term memory. In humans, a blow on the head can have a similar effect, as can electroshock treatment of the mentally ill. Some anaesthetics destroy all recollection of their administration. The witness to a crime could probably be 'silenced' if his memory storage were interrupted by some such means within an hour or so of the event.

Pacifying drugs. When a hunter is rounding up fierce or strong animals for zoo collections, a dart dosed with a tranquilliser or sedative can help him. Some pharmacologists fear that a dictatorship could put tranquillisers or similar drugs into a nation's water supply and thereby suppress any fierce resentment against the regime.

Research workers often compound the power of drugs with the pinpointing ability of the implanted electrode. They inject a chemical through a fine tube into a chosen part of the brain of an animal. By this means precise control becomes possible, which is very helpful for investigating brain mechanisms. It turns out, for example, that the same chemical injected at different parts of the brain can produce different effects; so can different chemicals injected at exactly the same point in the brain. One of the simplest and earliest discoveries was that salt water introduced into the 'thirst site' of an animal's brain (see page 49) forces him to drink. Fresh water at the same site makes a thirsty animal stop drinking.

From Princeton University, in 1970, Bartley Hoebel and his colleagues reported the control of the 'killing site' in the brain of a rat, by pinpoint introduction of a choice of drugs. In rats that were naturally peaceful and not inclined to attack mice sharing their cages, a small dose of a drug called carbachol, at the crucial site, prompted them to kill the mice. Carbachol stimulates activity in the relevant brain cells. Another drug, atropine, diminishes it and when rats that were natural killers were injected with atropine at the same site in the brain, they merely walked over to the mice and sniffed them.

From experiments like that, to what might be literally 'brainwashing' of humans with drugs, is a long step but it would be rash to say it could never be taken. Of the existing possibilities for mind control by drugs, the very simplest of those we have noted may be the most sinister – tranquillisers in the public water supply. Another scheme foreshadowed in fiction envisages the state as drug-pusher, exacting obedience in exchange for the daily 'trip'.

The more we learn about the workings of the brain, the more powerful will be the means of controlling the mind. The political risks should not be dismissed lightly. But it would be equally wrong to picture the world's brain researchers as Frankensteins intent upon turning man into a chemical robot. One might as well suggest that all doctors investigating the cause of disease are really in the pay of the military establishments that turn diseases into biological weapons. The new drugs have relieved untold human suffering in the psychiatric wards. Those who regard mind control with drugs as an affront to human integrity, even in severe mental illness, presumably would judge treatment by brain surgery or electrodes even

Drugs make wild animals easier to handle. Could the same principle be applied to 'wild' citizens?

Electrodes (left) can deliver an electrical stimulus to a selected region of the brain. The normal administration of a mind drug (middle) can produce chemical effects almost anywhere in the brain. The use of fine tubes or 'chemitrodes' (right) makes it possible to produce chemical effects in a selected region.

74

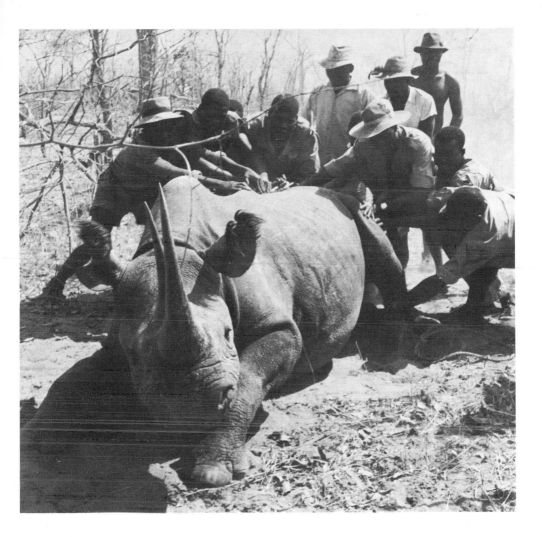

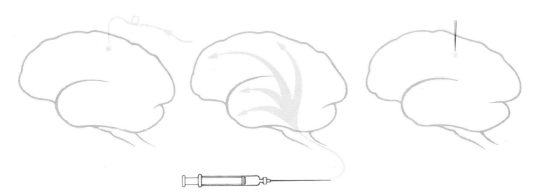

more harshly. One of the benefits of drugs has been to reduce the need for such procedures.

Among man's chief defences against would-be tyrants with hypodermics is his individuality. A mind drug can affect different people in very different ways, as everyone knows who has observed the consequences of alcohol at a party. A drug used successfully in treating seriously ill mental patients may have contradictory results in normal individuals. Patients suffering from depression have been known to take amphetamine to help them sleep! A given drug can have different effects on the same person at different times of day. Jonathan Cole of the US National Institutes of Health summed up the difficulty as follows: 'Even if one were only attempting to control the minds of a homogeneous group of psychiatric patients with a drug with which one had had considerable experience, the desired effect would not be produced in all patients, and one would not be able to plan specifically that any particular effect would be produced in a particular patient.'

Control without drugs

The psychiatrist, the propagandist and the mind-controller are out to change an individual's mind for his own good or for the sake of a communal or tyrannical cause. These three roles merge under those regimes which confine their opponents to mental hospitals, taking political aberration as a mark of insanity. So extreme a policy should be a warning to everyone. As techniques become more effective there is a danger that any kind of unconventional conduct might be systematically attacked by psychotherapy.

The more rigorous methods of mind control must be kept in perspective. All our minds are shaped from birth by information, advice, commands, promises and threats. Moreover, some of us are manifestly very sick in our heads and suffer untold grief for it; the psychiatrists' plain duty is to use any reasonable means to remake such minds. The famous issues of nature versus nurture and of the individual versus the community, which reach to the core of all politics and personal conduct, are better postponed until we have penetrated deeper into the machinery of the mind. Here we are concerned with the light shed on that machinery, and on human nature, by 'mechanical' aids to mind control.

Some techniques of brainwashing fall in this category, although they involve nothing like drugs or implanted electrodes. Stories told of the likely effectiveness of brainwashing are often exaggerated yet there is no denying human vulnerability to torture, mental as well as physical. One of the simplest and cruellest techniques is sensory deprivation – the denial of the normal inflow of information from the environment which is not merely interesting but essential for the proper functioning of the brain (see page 32).

Donald Hebb says, of the typical student who took part in his group's experiments of this kind at Montreal, that taking away the usual sights, sounds and bodily contacts could disturb his capacity for critical judgement, 'making him eager to listen to and believe any sort of preposterous nonsense'. Solitary confinement in a bare and silent cell is an ancient prelude to brainwashing. Sleep deprivation is another obvious and powerful technique for temporarily deranging an individual; political prisoners of our time have told of being woken by loud noises every quarter of an hour. Such treatment accelerates the effect of solitary confinement, as does confusing information – in the timing of meals, for example – which disorganises the victim's sense of time and place.

If a dog begins to recognise a bell as a signal of impending food, and then the food is witheld for increasingly long intervals, the dog will eventually break down completely, going into a state known as general inhibition. The same outcome occurs when a dog has been taught that a circle signals 'food' while an ellipse signals 'no food' and then the animal sees shapes that could be taken either as circles or ellipses. Even the most phlegmatic dog breaks down in these circumstances, if it is first physically exhausted by exercise or disease. Such procedures, from the classical experiments with dogs by Ivan Pavlov in Russia, give a rough scientific basis for further well-known techniques of mental assault on prisoners.

What is remarkable is not that forceful brainwashing is possible but that it can often be resisted. It is not very effective in implanting new opinions or false information in unwilling heads. Some people are very suggestible, whether or not they are ill-treated. Others, quite understandably, will agree to anything or confess to anything to escape further torture. When attention is individualised, the pressures can be made unendurable. But the results of a large-scale indoctrination effort of recent times – that of the Chinese on prisoners of the Korean war – were really quite unimpressive.

Americans were distressed that 13 per cent of their servicemen actively collaborated with their Chinese captors, but the reason seems to have been poor morale and discipline, and the unaccustomed experience of privation, rather than the ingenuity of the interrogators. Men who stood firm, giving no hint of co-operation whatever, were sometimes knocked about but their minds were left alone. A group of a hundred Turkish prisoners in Korea retained such discipline and comradeship that they completely resisted efforts in indoctrination.

Hypnosis is a more ritualised method of mind control and John Clark of Manchester University has developed a quasi-mechanical method for producing the hypnotic trance. His hypnotising machine is essentially a tape-recording of a voice going through the basic patter of the hypnotist. It is under the control of the subject himself, who has to press a button at

Hypnotism by machine. The subject listens to the tape recorder and presses a button to advance the tape to the next stage of the procedure. If he fails to press the button, the recent stage is repeated.

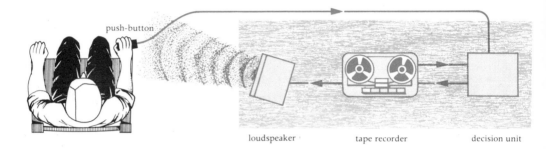

push-button

loudspeaker   tape recorder   decision unit

critical moments during the programme – for example, when his eyes are closed. Otherwise the previous part is automatically repeated as often as necessary. Superfluous parts of the ritual are stripped away, and all the subject looks at is a drawing-pin stuck in the wall.

This mechanisation is useful for research on hypnotism but it also tells us that, while the hypnotised state remains mysterious, there is nothing magical in the procedure for making the mind flip over into that state. It illustrates the immense power that words, even from a tape-recorder, can exert over the human mind, though hypnotism may also be possible without the use of words. While watching the hypnotist Jean-Martin Charcot at work in Paris, Sigmund Freud first suspected the existence of the unconscious mind, but since then hypnotism has figured only in a minor way in psychiatry and research.

What can be accomplished by the hypnotist? Demonstrations of robot-like response to commands, or of suggested immunity to pain, fall far short of enduring control of the conscious mind. No one is likely to do anything important as a result of hypnosis that he would not otherwise willingly do. Even the claims that, under hypnosis, a person can recall in detail long-forgotten experiences of his childhood become

78   doubtful, when it turns out that much of the information is

invented and the rest would be likely to be remembered anyway. Hypnosis may be useful, nevertheless, for digging out ordinary memories repressed in a mental patient.

As a technique of mind control, the weakness of hypnotism is that the unwilling subject can nearly always resist it. On the other hand, an important practical conclusion from studies of hypnotism is that some people – about one in twenty – are exceptionally prone to hypnosis and other suggestions. Stephen Black of London reported that most of the people he interviewed who had seen flying saucers fell into this category of deep-trance hypnotic subjects. Elements of the hypnotist's art may be adopted by priests and orators, to some effect.

Anyone who is justifiably worried by some of the possibilities of mind control rehearsed in the foregoing pages has already gone a long way towards conceding that the human brain and mind are scarcely distinguishable. If a wire in the brain can give one man sublime pleasure, while a drug radically alters the thoughts and actions of another conscious mind, and a tape-recorder is persuading a third man that his arm is rigid, what is the human mind except a machine – the machine we know as the brain?

We need not say merely a machine: the brain is an amazing machine of immense power. The chief consequence of mind control with electrodes and drugs may lie, not in any direct use or misuse, but in the fact that it is possible and in the long-term influence of this knowledge. It is humbling knowledge, certainly, but need not be humiliating. As for the vulnerability of our minds to physical or psychological control by external agents, nothing yet discovered in the way of new techniques detracts from the exclamation of defiance by the nineteenth-century Russian author, Fyodor Dostoevsky: 'Out of sheer ingratitude man will play you a dirty trick, just to prove that men are still men and not the keys of a piano.'

There remains another possible innuendo, from the experiments and theories described in the previous chapters, that the mind of the individual may be the helpless prisoner of the natural chemistry of the body. If our awakening to consciousness is a chemical process, if our attention is governed by the flickering activity of brain cells, if changes in our lines of thought from day to day are markedly influenced by the hormones circulating in our blood, what price our mental powers? But to be so pessimistic about mind control, whether the influence originates within or outside the body, is to underestimate human will and the way mental processes can override the most importunate chemistry of the body.

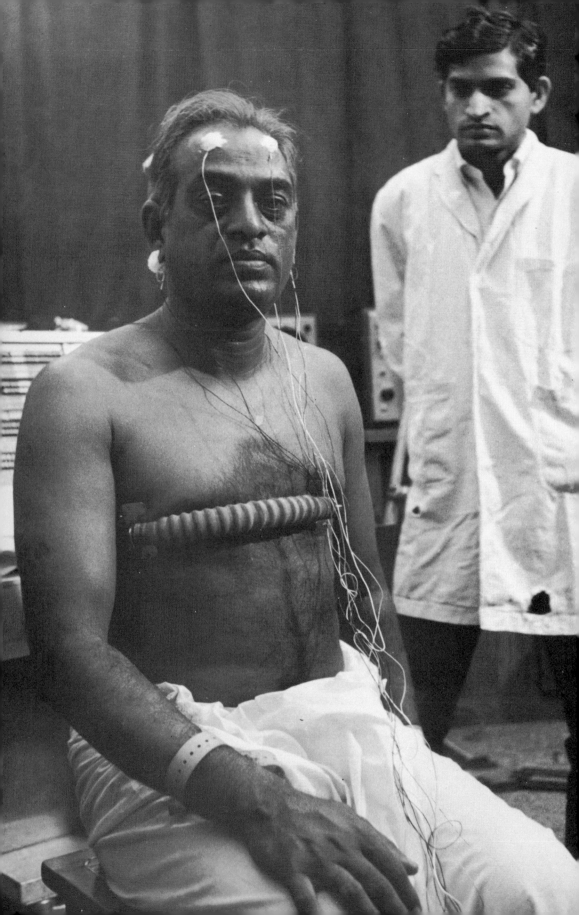

5

An Inward Spaceflight

The very recent discovery that the conscious mind has astonishing control over basic bodily functions, hitherto thought to be beyond its reach, promises to alter our view of human nature. Meanwhile it is being put to practical use in experimental treatment of disorders such as high blood pressure.

Ramanand Yogi, 'wired up' in preparation for a test of his ability to reduce his body's demand for oxygen.

On 4 March 1970, a remarkable experiment took place in a laboratory in New Delhi. It had been intended as a repetition, in front of a BBC film camera, of an earlier experiment. As it turned out, it gave new results so dramatic that word leaked out to Indira Gandhi, the Indian prime minister, and the minister of health came hurrying around to see what was going on at the All-India Institute of Medical Sciences.

These were the days of *Apollo* and of the expansion of the human will into a cosmic playground. Less than a year before this adventure in Delhi, the first men had stepped on the surface of the moon; only a few weeks after it, the crippled *Apollo 13* made its lucky return to earth. But the capsule in Bal Krishan Anand's physiological laboratory was not designed to move. The flight the man inside it was making was a strange one, into the very depths of his own being. His mental journey afforded the most striking authentication yet of the power of the mind to dominate the body.

Ramanand Yogi, 46 years old, from Hyderabad in the Telugu-speaking area of India, was the performer. At the age of 18 he had separated from his young wife and daughter to devote himself to Yoga. Largely by self-instruction he became very accomplished, a 'raj yogi', but unlike most of those very rare individuals he did not isolate himself from the world. By 1951 he claimed to be able to stay alive for 28 days when buried underground. Even allowing for seepage of gases through the soil, such a feat would suggest that he had to survive on considerably less oxygen than a normal person.

This was one of the points that Anand and his colleague G. S. Chhina were anxious to look into when, in 1959, Ramanand Yogi had agreed to submit to their tests. Anand is a distinguished brain researcher and a council member of the International

Brain Research Organisation. In 1951, while working at Yale University, he had been co-discoverer of the 'feeding sites' in the brain. Neither he nor his staff would be readily taken in by any deception.

Indeed, in one of their early series of tests of Ramanand and some other yogis, Anand and Chhina quickly cleared up a mystery that had baffled competent doctors for years: the apparent ability of some yogis to 'stop their hearts' so that they seemed to be dead. The recording instruments of Anand's physiology department revealed how the trick was done.

The yogis would hold their breath and contract the muscles of their chest and abdomen to build up pressure in the chest. They could thereby reduce the flow of blood sufficiently to make the action of the heart almost inaudible in a stethoscope, and the pulse in the wrist very weak. But, so far from stopping, the heart actually speeded up during this manoeuvre – which the yogis could sustain for only 10 to 20 seconds.

In a spirit of intelligent scepticism, therefore, and with no special interest in the religious aspects of Yoga, the Indian medical scientists examined the physical powers exhibited by the yogis during meditation. But they began to find effects that could not be explained away and which flouted a principle of modern brain theory – namely that basic functions within the body are beyond voluntary control. In one case, a yogi was able to slow down (not to stop) his heart at will. Another yogi was

The recorder monitors the brain rhythms, heart rate and breathing of a yogi sealed in an airtight box.

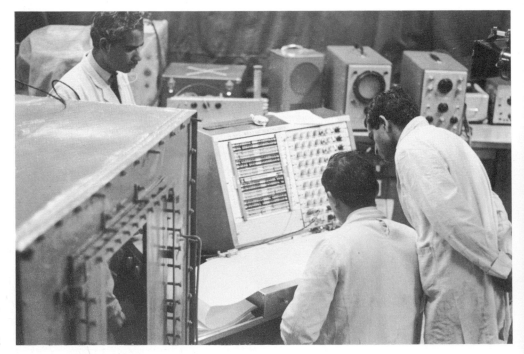

able to make himself sweat at his forehead only. These accomplishments were less dramatic than the claims of stopping the heart but they were very telling from a theoretical point of view.

The big surprise came when Anand, Chhina and Baldev Singh persuaded Ramanand Yogi to go into an airtight box in their laboratory. The aim was to cast light on the yogi's claim that he could survive prolonged burial. A metal box was prepared, six feet long by four feet square, with an airtight entry port, glass for observation and provision for drawing off air samples from time to time. The volume of the yogi, his mattress

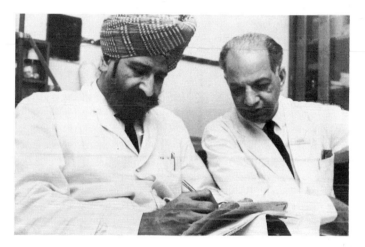

G. S. Chhina computes the yogi's oxygen consumption during the experiment. B. K. Anand looks on.

and everything else inside was taken into account in computing the volume of air available. The yogi was 'wired up' to record his heart rate, breathing rate, body temperature and brain waves.

The first experiment was not successful. Ramanand Yogi lit a candle inside the box, which made nonsense of the attempts to measure his own oxygen intake. A week later, everyone tried again – this time with no candle. The yogi stayed in the box for ten hours, in a trance. Every half-hour a sample of air was drawn off from the interior of the box. Anand, Chhina and Singh saw with some incredulity that the oxygen content of the box was falling, and the carbon-dioxide level rising, more slowly than they ought to be doing.

They had previously measured Ramanand's oxygen requirements at rest but not meditating and had calculated a lowest figure for what is known as basal metabolism – the least rate of expenditure of energy (and oxygen) which is necessary for the maintenance of the life of the body even during complete inactivity. To go below this rate, by intention, would be like willing your hair to grow more slowly. At stake were the most 83 basic processes of sustenance and repair within the body. And yet these were precisely what the yogi overruled.

Ramanand's brain waves showed the relaxed drowsiness of meditation. His heart and breathing were slow and calm until towards the end of the experiment, when even he could no longer suppress the reaction to incipient suffocation with carbon dioxide. Although the temperature of the box was held steady at 27° C. (80·6° F.), the yogi was feverish for most of the experiment, with a body temperature of 39° C. (102·2° F.). Over the ten-hour period as a whole, Ramanand consumed oxygen to the extent of only 70 per cent of that predicted from his basal metabolic rate. More strikingly, during the middle hours he was consuming oxygen at a rate of half the theoretical minimum.

Anand and his colleagues published the results of this and other yogi experiments in 1961. In spite of their sharp contradictions of an accepted theory of how the brain worked, the results were almost wholly ignored outside India. Nine years later, as we shall see, experiments in the United States had sapped the theory until it collapsed. It then seemed only fair, in reporting this development, to go back to the laboratory in New Delhi where the advance had been anticipated. At our

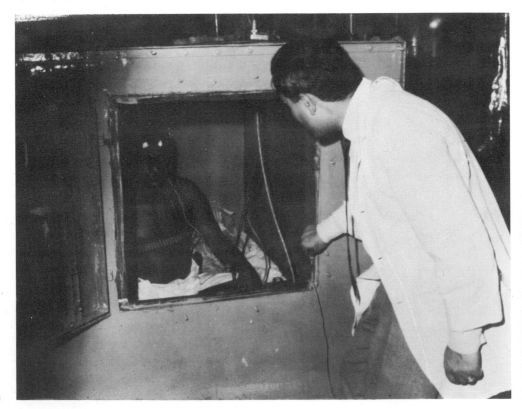

request, for the television programme, Ramanand Yogi, Professor Anand and Dr Chhina all agreed to re-enact the experiment in the airtight box.

Mind over matter

In the 1970 experiment in New Delhi, Ramanand stayed in the airtight box for less than six hours, but Anand had always stressed that the aim was not a test of endurance. The camera rolled as the yogi said his prayers before entering the box. All the paraphernalia of instrumentation were fitted to his head and half-naked body. Then the glass door of the box was bolted on to its seals. The yogi was alone with his limited air supply and with a buzzer he could sound if he wanted to be released. While the laboratory staff tended their instruments, Ramanand began his inward journey of meditation.

From the start, the experiment went differently. The theoretical minimum for the yogi's oxygen consumption, at the basal metabolic rate, had been calculated at about 9·7 litres per half-hour. In the experiment ten years before, the rate was exceeded during the first half-hour. But on this occasion Ramanand was away more quickly. He consumed only 6·8 litres of oxygen in

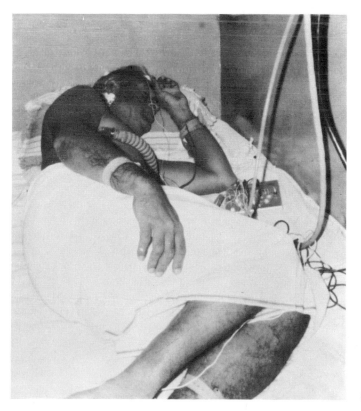

Ramanand Yogi at New Delhi, March 1970, in the airtight box in which he made his 'inward spaceflight'. In his trance (right) he has cut his oxygen requirements to one quarter of the minimum rate thought theoretically to be possible.

the first half-hour, and during the second half-hour he was down to 4·7 litres of oxygen. Ninety minutes later he was still hovering around that level – about half the theoretical minimum, much the same as he attained in the earlier experiments.

Then the sixth air sample was taken for analysis, three hours into the experiment. The analysis showed very little reduction in oxygen, or increase in carbon dioxide, compared with the previous sample. So small was the change, in fact, that Ramanand's consumption in the previous half-hour worked out at only 2·3 litres of oxygen. Anand and Chhina, the chief experimenters, were astonished as they checked the figures. The wires from the yogi's scalp brought evidence of very rhythmic electrical activity of the half-sleeping state; his heartbeats and breathing were slow but sure, despite the rising level of carbon dioxide in his air. Had some error of measurement been made?

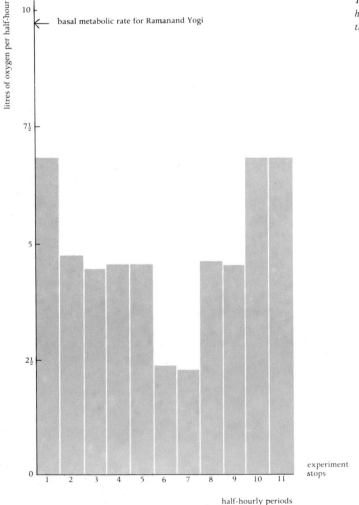

The yogi's oxygen consumption in half-hourly periods during the experiment of 4 March 1970.

Everyone waited expectantly for the next half-hourly sample and its analysis. When it came, it showed an oxygen consumption of 2·2 litres. Ramanand Yogi had voluntarily knocked his requirement down to one quarter of the minimum supposed necessary for the maintenance of life. The *Bhagavad-Gita,* holy book of the yogis, remarks aptly:

As a blazing fire turns fuel to ashes,
so does the fire of knowledge turn all actions into ashes.

Ramanand failed to keep down to this level for long. The inexorable increase in carbon dioxide inside the box made it impossible for him to stay in so deep a trance. During the next two hours his oxygen consumption rose by steps. Signs of disturbance began to show on the monitoring instruments. Then, quite suddenly, Ramanand sounded the alarm buzzer.

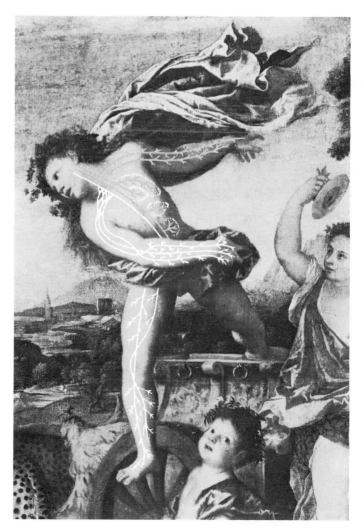

Orthodox divisions of the nervous system are shown schematically. The motor nervous system (white) governs gross bodily movements and speech. The autonomic nervous system (colour) acts on internal organs, blood vessels, etc. It was wrongly thought to be beyond direct conscious control. It has two divisions: the sympathetic and parasympathetic systems which tend to be contradictory in their effects. The sensory nerves which bring information to the brain from all parts of the body are not shown. (Modified detail from Titian's Bacchus and Ariadne*)*

For a fevered minute or so the laboratory staff wrestled to loosen the bolts that separated the yogi from the outside air. When at last he emerged he was complaining of a very painful ear, caused by a detector fixed to it. But he was alive and generally well, despite the fact that, three hours previously, he had brought the 'essential' metabolism of his body nearly to a halt.

What was so upsetting for orthodox Western medicine and brain research, about such investigations of the control of internal bodily functions? Perhaps the quickest way to show it is to quote from *Black's Medical Dictionary* (1967 edition):

> AUTONOMIC NERVOUS SYSTEM is the term applied to that part of the nervous system which regulates the functions of some of the internal organs independently of the will power . . . .

The belief, dating from the nineteenth century, was that human beings could consciously control their external (skeletal) muscles and very little else. Heart-beat, blood pressure, skin temperature and the activity of the glands – all such housekeeping operations of the body were held to be almost entirely beyond the reach of the conscious mind; hence the name for the networks responsible for these matters, the 'autonomic', or self-governing, nervous system. Belief in its autonomy persisted despite evidence to the contrary. With it went the view that the emotions, being enmeshed with the internal state of the body, were beyond the full control of reason.

Part of the contrary evidence was there for all to see – not tucked away in laboratories or in the retreats of the Indian holy men, but highly conspicuous on theatre stages and on cinema and television screens. When an accomplished actor shows emotion, he is not merely making the right noises and grimaces. Some actors actually feel angry or sad or loving, to just the degree necessary for a convincing but controlled performance, after the methods of one of the most influential teachers of acting, Konstantin Stanislavsky of Moscow. That is an indirect way of controlling the glandular responses. Other actors claim to produce tears, blushing and the like, without needing to 'feel that way' to obtain the effect. This is a truer sign of direct control and such claims need no longer be doubted.

Stanislavsky required his actors to learn to think appropriate thoughts at each moment on the stage, which would evoke the right feelings. But the student was also expected to do strenuous mental exercises – a kind of purposeful meditation. And, when conscious preparation had reached its limit, Stanis-

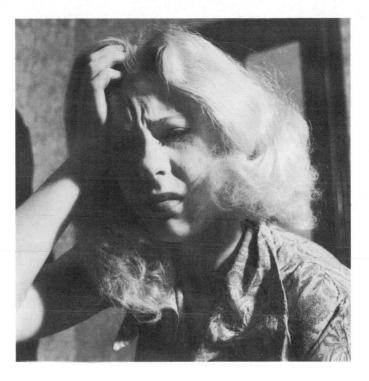

Some accomplished actors claim to produce tears at will without even feeling sad. If so, they are exerting direct conscious control over the so-called autonomic nervous system.

lavsky commended to his pupils the practical advice offered by the yogis of India. The actor should go on and fortify his internal state, so that 'inspiration' might step out from the conscious mind. Stanislavsky's methods have been largely superseded in Western drama schools but conscious control, either of feelings or of the symptoms of feelings, remains an everyday ingredient of good acting.

Other clues to conscious influences on the internal state of the body came from brain studies, particularly from known nerve links between internal organs and the roof of the brain. Anand's interest in yogis was not casually inspired; he was primarily a student of the brain systems serving drive and emotion and he knew of interplay between these systems and higher regions of the brain. But the delusion about the autonomy of the autonomic nervous system might have persisted till now if a leading American psychologist had not staked his high reputation on the issue – Neal Miller, now at the Rockefeller University, New York City.

Prejudice confounded

Miller was at Yale University when he turned his efforts, at the end of the 1950s, to training animals to control their autonomic nervous systems. The absurdity of his enterprise was so apparent that he had extreme difficulty in persuading even his own students to help him in the experimental work. And when paid assistants were assigned to it, as Miller recalls, 'their attempts were so half-hearted that it soon became more economical to let them work on some other problem . . . .' Other snags were technical. It was hard to insulate internal responses, such as heart rate, from the indirect effects of voluntary muscular activity – if you sprint, your heart will speed up. Also, the actual rewards given to animals during training could excite them in ways unintended in the experiment.

Some academic psychologists, it seems to me, would refuse to believe that human beings had a sex life, unless it were first demonstrated in the laboratory rat. By the 1960s, animalism had replaced animism to such a degree that all the human evidence, of yogis or actors, counted for little. If control of the autonomic nervous system was to be believed at all, rats had to show it. And so they did, in a long and eventually incontestable series of experiments by Neal Miller and his colleagues. Miller's own reason for preferring rats to humans was technical rather than ideological: the potentially confusing activities of muscles were to be prevented by a paralysing drug, curare.

As it happened, dogs were the animals that figured in the earliest of Miller's experiments which gave clear-cut results. It was a bold variation of Pavlov's classical conditioning of

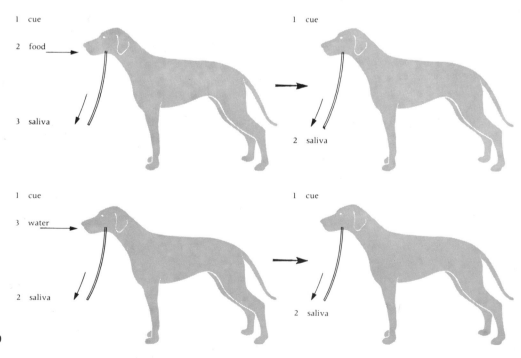

salivation and nothing could have been more apt, in view of the nature of the theory at issue. Pavlov's famous demonstration (1903) of the so-called conditioned reflex involved a dog whose mouth would water at the sound of a bell because, during training, the bell had usually just preceded the presentation of food. The glands producing saliva are controlled by the autonomic nervous system.

In the 1930s, Polish and American psychologists codified the second great means of conditioning animal behaviour – by reward or punishment after the animal has performed or has failed to perform a certain act. After some exploratory experiments by Burrhus F. Skinner, it was quickly accepted that this operant conditioning or instrumental learning was ineffective in influencing the autonomic nervous system. Control pecking or running, yes; salivation or heart-rate, no. Thus did the psychologists carry over, into learning theory, the nineteenth-century dichotomy of the neurologists. Neal Miller never accepted the distinction between the two kinds of learning.

Working with Alfredo Carmona, Miller trained a group of dogs to increase their spontaneous salivation – measured in drops per minute – simply by rewarding them with a drink of water whenever they did so. They arranged, of course, that the dogs were suitably thirsty at the training sessions. And, in case anyone should say that the water itself promoted salivation, they trained another group of dogs to salivate *less*, using the same reward. After daily training sessions for about five weeks, the first group of dogs had doubled their spontaneous mouth-watering and the second group had halved it.

A wide variety of experiments with rats followed. The rats were temporarily paralysed with curare and artificial respiration kept them alive. Miller and his colleagues found that, in these unlikely circumstances, the rats learned to control their autonomic activities much more rapidly than did the dogs in the saliva experiment. The reward given was electric stimulation of a 'pleasure site' in the brain. When tested afterwards without curare, the rats had retained the habits so learned. The experimenters produced large increases or decreases, at will, in the following activities of the body previously thought to be beyond such control:

heart rate,
blood pressure,
constriction of the blood vessels in the tail, the ears or the
    stomach,
rate of contractions in the intestine,
rate of formation of urine.

Pavlov's 'conditioned reflex' (upper diagram) controls the production of saliva in a dog's mouth after training with food, which itself provokes salivation. Eventually the bell associated with food is sufficient to cause salivation. Miller's 'instrumental learning' (lower diagram) controls the production of saliva simply by rewarding the animal with water for success in changing it. Salivation can be increased or decreased by this procedure, showing that the change is not an uncontrolled response to the water.

91

Some checking experiments eliminated the possibility that processes within the body were interfering with one another or that the responses in the experiments were side-effects of some more conventional response. According to the traditional view, one large part of the autonomic nervous system worked to raise heart-rate, reduce bowel contraction and produce a whole range of other effects, in unison, while another part reversed all its effects, again in unison.

Miller showed that rats learning to change their heart rate did not change their rates of bowel contractions; and vice versa. The control was as specific as the closing of an eye or the raising of a leg.

By the summer of 1969, when the International Congress of Psychology met in London, Neal Miller was able to present overwhelming evidence for a 'radical reorientation of thinking'. From now on, his message ran, we must think of the actions of the glands and internal organs, concealed inside the body, in exactly the same way as we think of the actions of the muscles producing easily observable movement. The nervous system governing the former is not in any fundamental sense inferior to that governing the latter. What follows from this radical reorientation?

Balance redressed

In 1970, patients with high blood pressure were helping in initial trials, in a New York hospital, of a possible new form of treatment – learning to reduce their own blood pressure just

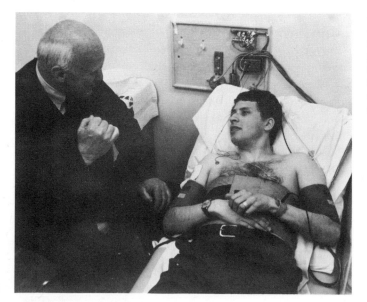

Neal Miller with a volunteer at the Bellevue Hospital, New York, who is to learn to control his blood pressure, listening for a signal that tells of success. Mastery of the internal organs and glands does not necessarily require elaborate training, as in Yoga.

by taking thought. Neal Miller had already participated in medical tests of the control of the human autonomic nervous system, in two people with racing hearts (tachycardia) who were able to learn to slow them down. The benefits seemed to persist after the training finished. In another therapeutic trial, Miller and his colleagues had some success in training epileptic patients to suppress the abnormal electric activity in the brain which is characteristic of their condition.

The procedure is very simple indeed. The patient lies relaxed in the lab. He is fitted with an instrument for measuring his blood pressure, or whatever else he is supposed to be controlling. Whenever he manages to change it in the right direction and to the required degree, he hears a tone which tells him of his progress. Gone are the elaborate ritual practices of Yoga; these may serve some intellectual purpose among the devotees but they are not needed for the control of the autonomic nervous system. Miller had also dismissed the scheme adopted by David Shapiro and his colleagues of the Harvard Medical School who, in the first of such experiments in humans, rewarded volunteers with projected slides – typically, nudes from *Playboy* magazine – as they achieved a measure of control of their internal organs. In Miller's opinion, a signal of success is all the reward that a human being requires.

But he would like to be able to advise patients more precisely on how to think about what they are supposed to be achieving. He likens their task to that of a blindfold golfer. Certainly, in Miller's set-up, human beings can be trained to control a function without knowing what it is, or in what direction they are supposed to be changing it. But learning may be faster and more durable if patients have a clearer sense of what they are doing.

He is also concerned about the scope for unconscious or even conscious cheating by a patient who might, for example, alter his breathing rate to fake a measure of control of internal organs. These technical questions aside, Miller is optimistic about widening the medical purposes that the training procedure can serve. Possibilities that he has in mind range from attempting the control of asthma to encouraging, in patients with insomnia, the electric brain rhythms of the kind that occur during sleep. Other investigators have already trained patients to improve the rhythms of their hearts.

Striking though they are, these direct medical uses of learning to control the internal functions of the body may be almost the least of the consequences of the discovery (*pace* the yogis) that such control is possible. We must expect a revolution in medicine, not necessarily in the sense that we shall learn to control measles by listening for a tone, but because the interaction between mind and body must from now on be taken very much more seriously as a cause or influence in disease.

'Psychosomatic' medicine, concerned with the mental factors in disease, seemed a dubious enterprise in the first half of this century. One reason was the theoretical gulf separating the conscious mind and the autonomic nervous system which operated internally in the body. Traditional medicine allowed that a person might die 'of a broken heart'. When nineteenth-century authors killed off their unhappy heroines with tuberculosis they were drawing on all-too-familiar medical and lay experience of their time. Modern medical science, with its aptitude for discovering the microbe or the biochemical defect directly responsible for disease, tended to push mental factors into the background – not unjustifiably, in practical terms, because tuberculosis, for example, is almost conquered in the richer nations of the world.

Growing concern about bodily diseases that were apparently promoted by the psychological stresses of modern urban life aided a recent revival of psychosomatic medicine. Stephen Black of London has summarised the evidence for psychological effects in allergies, ranging from asthma to dermatitis, and in other conditions. Black also cites strange results achieved with suggestion under hypnosis, such as the suggestion that warts should disappear from one side of a patient's body and not from the other – which reportedly worked in nine cases out of ten. But psychosomatic medicine has remained controversial and comparatively few medical men have engaged in it conspicuously. That situation can hardly endure, in the light of the discoveries of Anand and Miller. The brain has an even more direct effect on the internal actions of the body than those doctors supposed.

A unification of medicine is due, which fully accepts the importance both of mental factors in physical disease and of physical factors in mental disease. Drugs can produce and possibly discourage the frank madness characteristic of schizophrenia. Mental processes can encourage and possibly discourage bodily malfunction, such as heart disease. It becomes possible also to envisage training the mind to alter bodily chemistry so as to relieve mental disease. A new and sensible variant of 'faith' healing may be on its way. All that can be said with confidence is that a whole new area of medical research is opened up by the control of the autonomic nervous system. The results of that research cannot really be anticipated, although they are likely to be exciting.

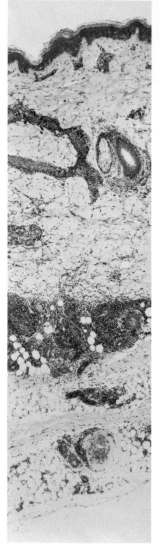

The mind can affect the human body's defences against foreign material. Here, shown at a magnification of × 45, is a section of skin swollen in the Mantoux test for previous tuberculosis infection.

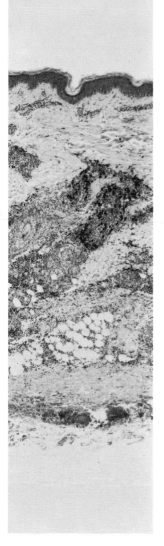

Surpassing even these open-ended medical implications in importance is what the discovery tells us about human nature in everyday life, far from the hospital or the psychiatric clinic. Control of the autonomic nervous system redresses the balance against everything stated in the earlier chapters concerning the vulnerability of the human mind to physical and chemical influences.

Our awakening and level of excitement depend, as we have seen, upon physical and chemical activity sweeping up from the brain stem. Our drives and emotions are similarly engineered, with the assistance of hormones coursing through the body, or the prevailing state of the heart and blood pressure. With man-made drugs and implanted wires the processes of mind are open to manipulation. On such evidence it would be easy to arrive at a low opinion of man – to see ourselves as highly emotional robots entirely at the mercy of switches that operate capriciously below the level of consciousness.

So long as there was a lack of symmetry, so long as the hormones and the heart could influence the conscious mind but the mind was not allowed directly to influence the hormones and the heart, that self-denigration was rather plausible. It ceases to be so now that the two-way process is restored. Chemistry in the form of sex hormone or LSD may sometimes overwhelm the mind, but the mind can also dominate chemistry – even to the staggering degree achieved by Ramanand Yogi during his inward spaceflight in the airtight box.

Both processes testify to the essentially physical nature of mind and its intimate involvement with the body, but the latter process is especially healing for our self-respect. It supplies a satisfactory note on which to end this part of the book, as we redirect our search for the mind into the intricate labyrinths in the roof of the brain.

No swelling in the skin of the same person, after suggestion under hypnosis that the reaction to the test should be negative. At the cellular level, the reaction is unaltered. (Photomicrographs by Janet Niven)

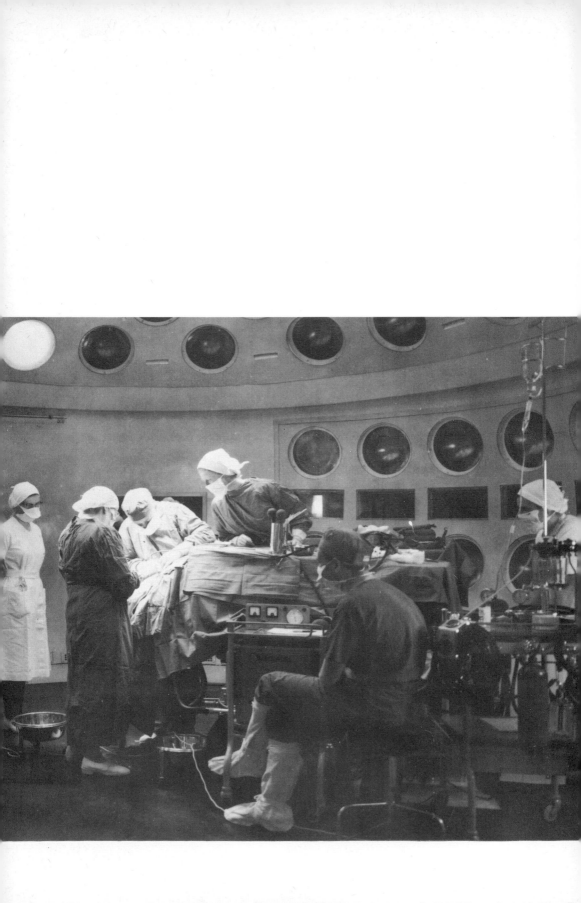

6

Bullet in the Brain

Those unfortunate humans who lose certain powers, because of injury or disease in the brain, supply much of our knowledge of how various functions of mental life are shared out between the different regions. Although some functions and some brain regions remain mysterious, others are already well mapped.

Men in war employ their brains to contrive to shoot metal into the brains of other men. In 1943, while the armies of Hitler and Stalin were locked in the bloodiest campaigns of the Second World War, among those gravely wounded was a brave and bright young officer of the Red Army, Lev Zassetsky. Z, as we shall call him, had a part of his head shot away, on the left and

In Edinburgh's Western General Hospital, a modern theatre for brain operations (left). In Moscow's Burdenko Institute, Alexander Luria tests his war-wounded patient Z (right). The damage to Z's brain (below) left him confused about the difference between 'above' and 'beneath'.

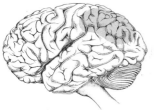

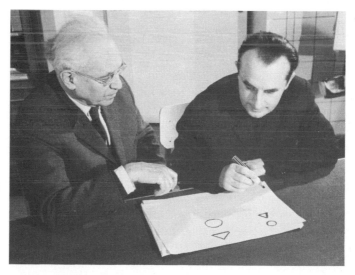

towards the back. His personality was not changed nor his courage impaired, which was just as well because his war has lasted the rest of his life as he has struggled with the damage to his mind.

His vision was affected and he lost his ordinary ability to read and write. But he was fortunate enough to come under the care of Alexander Luria of Moscow, one of the world's leading specialists on the mental effects of brain damage. Luria found that Z could still sign his name. In other words he could write 97 when he did not attempt to work out how to form the letters and words. With great effort, using a brain mechanism different from that involved in normal writing, Z learned to write again. Over 25 years, leading the quiet life of a war pensioner, he has written a manuscript of 3,000 pages of eloquent autobiography. Here is an extract from his introduction (translated by Michael Glenny):

> Many people, I know, discuss cosmic space and how our earth is no more than a tiny particle in the infinite universe, and now they are talking seriously of flight to the nearer planets of the solar system. Yet the flight of bullets, shrapnel, shells or bombs which splinter and fly into a man's head, poisoning and scorching his brain, crippling his memory, sight, hearing, consciousness – this is now regarded as something normal and easily dealt with. But is it? If so, then why am I sick, why doesn't my memory function, why have I not regained my sight, why is there a constant noise in my aching head, why can't I hear or understand human speech properly? It is an appalling task to start again at the beginning and relearn the world which I lost when I was wounded, to piece it together again from tiny separate fragments into a single whole.

Basic aspects of the brain as an instrument of survival have occupied the preceding chapters; in particular the interplay of arousal, attention and emotion. Only latterly, in seeing the yogi-like dominance of these basic processes by the conscious mind, did we really begin to invoke the higher abilities that lie in the human brain. In this next part of the book, we take the alert brain and look within it for the faculties we may recognise as the mind in action.

We have to grasp at two ends of the scale of mechanisms. On the one hand there is the life-size brain in all its complexity, in which we can see some allocation and integration of mental systems. The present chapter introduces this theme. At the other end of the scale are microscopic and sub-microscopic processes too small for the eye to observe without powerful instruments. They involve individual, electrically active brain cells and the chemical links between them. In the middle of the scale – where cells become systems – there is a vast gap in present-day possibilities of explanation, but one or two parts of the brain are beginning to disclose the exquisite details of their organisation.

Luria's patient Z, in his hard-won ability to write, already illustrates two important features of the distribution of mental powers through the brain. First, the brain has surprising ability to withstand damage, to recuperate from it, and to improvise methods of functioning when normal powers have been lost. Luria describes Z as possessing 'an artificial mind'. Secondly, in a function like handwriting, several different systems take part, which are differently located; as a result, damage to one of them can leave the others unimpaired. Closer examination of Z shows a third feature of brain organisation: that one region of the brain can serve several, apparently quite different, functions.

If you were to ask Z to tell you the way to a particular street, or to draw a map, he would be likely to confuse left and right, or east and west. Requested by Luria to draw a circle above a triangle, Z struggles to work out the meaning of 'above' and which figure goes where. 'Is it true that a fly is bigger than an elephant?' or 'Are your brother's father and your father's brother the same person?' – questions like these are thoroughly perplexing for Z, even though he has begun, with his 'artificial mind', to contrive ways of reasoning his way towards the answers.

A pattern emerges: Z has lost the use of the part of the brain which enables a man to visualise the spatial or diagrammatic relationships between objects. This faculty serves many tasks that apparently have nothing to do with seeing. Most people probably use it when doing mental arithmetic (visualising the numbers laid out in a pattern) or when understanding a complex sentence (like this one you are reading now). Z, at any rate, has difficulties both with calculation and with grammar.

Hans-Lukas Teuber of the Massachusetts Institute of Technology tells of a similar case: a 17-year-old American serviceman in Korea with a hole in his head 'big enough to admit a fist'. He wandered in no-man's-land for three days, quite aimlessly. These unfortunate soldiers illustrate what surgeons have long known: that the so-called parietal lobes, high on the side of the brain, are the repository of the human sense of orientation. A person injured in a parietal lobe may have at least temporary problems in dressing himself; he is likely to have persistent difficulty with diagrams and mazes. The parietal lobes evidently pool information acquired by sight, hearing, touch and from the inner sensors of the body, to make internal maps showing how the world is laid out and how the body stands in relation to the world. The normal thinking brain probably draws on the power of the parietal lobes to make imaginary diagrams.

Z is one case among many thousands. Moscow's Burdenko Institute is only one of the big brain clinics around the world where surgeons and psychologists struggle to save life, mental and physical. The effects of brain damage, whether due to war, accident, illness or calculated excision by the surgeon, are the prime source of information about what goes on inside the head. The knowledge accumulated over many years helps the treatment and rehabilitation of each patient. It also illuminates the organisation of the normal, uninjured human brain. There are not many other sources of information.

Maps of mentality

Fyodor Dostoevsky described, in *The Idiot*, the feelings of an epileptic about to have a fit:

> . . . suddenly in the midst of sadness, spiritual darkness and oppression, there seemed at moments a flash of light in his brain, and with extraordinary impetus all his vital forces suddenly began working at their highest tension. The sense of life, the consciousness of self, were multiplied ten times at these moments which passed like a flash of lightning. His mind and his heart were flooded with extraordinary light; all his uneasiness, all his doubts, all his anxieties were relieved at once; they were all merged in a lofty calm, full of serene, harmonious joy and hope. But these moments, these flashes, were only the prelude of that final second (it was never more than a second) with which the fit began. That second was, of course, unendurable.

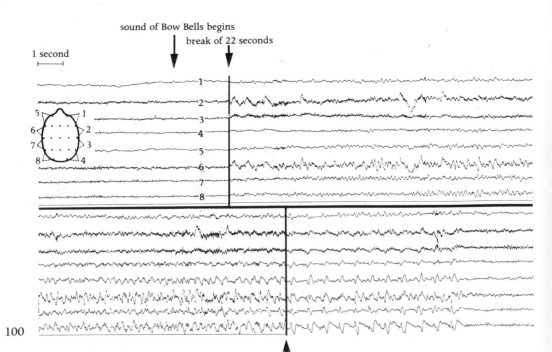

sound of Bow Bells begins

break of 22 seconds

1 second

break of 10 seconds

100

Dostoevsky did not have this by hearsay; he himself suffered from epilepsy. From this description and other, non-fictional accounts that he gave, it has since been deduced at which point in his brain his fits began. The ancients sometimes regarded epilepsy with religious awe. It is still an alarming, occasionally dangerous, state, for the victim and onlooker alike, but we now know that it is an electric storm in the brain, which can start from one region and spread to neighbouring regions. During the attack, the patient is unconscious, but his sensations immediately before it begins indicate the focal point – often an injured part of the brain.

Dostoevsky's fits evidently originated inside his left temple, in the temporal lobe of the roof of the brain, a region where mechanisms of joy and terror are curiously interleaved. For other epileptics, the prelude, or 'aura', can be quite different (an imagined smell, a peculiar feeling in the arm, a vision) depending on locality. The course of the attack, as the storm spreads, gives clues about what functions lie adjacent in the brain. If, for example, the patient contorts his face or jerks his limbs about it means that the storm has swept into the regions of the brain subserving movement.

A century ago the British neurologist Hughlings Jackson was making deductions from 'the march of the fit' which helped to put him far ahead of his time in the description of brain function. Jackson did not share the opportunity of twentieth-century brain surgeons using local anaesthetics, who began working with the human skull open and the patient awake. It then became possible gently to explore the surface of the living brain with electrodes, while the patient reported his experiences at each stimulation. After beginnings in Germany and the USA, this procedure became, in the hands of Wilder Penfield of Montreal, a technique of great value.

Penfield was able, in certain cases of severe epilepsy, to stimulate various points of the brain until a point was found where the patient said he felt just as he did at the onset of a fit. Removing a little of the brain around that point would usually cure or moderate the epilepsy. In the course of such explorations, Penfield and his followers have built up diagrams of the organisation of the exposed surface of the brain. For treatment and incidental mapping of regions hidden from view, surgeons nowadays use very precise 'aiming' equipment for guiding wires through the delicate upper layers to predetermined points deep in the brain.

Detailed maps can be drawn of the human brain, based upon all these effects of brain damage, of epilepsy, and of electrical stimulation, and supplemented by animal studies. The maps

The electric storm of epilepsy is shown by a brain-wave (EEG) recording in an unusual case – an elderly man in whom the seizure is provoked only by the sound of London's Bow Bells. The diagram of the head shows the pick-ups corresponding to the eight traces of fluctuating voltage. Strong rhythms appearing in the temporal regions on the left side (traces 6 to 8) grow in intensity. The storm ends quite suddenly. (Record from Kiloh and Osselton) need to be treated with a little caution. Many functions involve several regions of the brain, organised as interconnected systems rather than a single entity. Other functions seem indifferent to locality and are easily restored if brain damage is not too widespread. And the brain's organisation goes down to a very small scale, with the interconnection of individual brain cells; the rather gross effects here described cannot show such detail.

The fake science of the phrenologists, who offer to deduce character and fate by feeling the bumps and hollows in the skull, gives further reason for caution. In the past, some very fanciful maps of the brain have been drawn, allotting regions to thrift, to love of animals, to love of wine, and so on. The modern brain explorer tries to find a middle path between excessively exact localisation of brain function and the contradictory opinion that was fashionable earlier in this century, that the brain always operated as a single unit.

To weary the reader with a mass of detailed information about the mapping of the brain would be no more appropriate than to describe a ship by naming all the crew. The accompanying illustrations should convey the general idea – that mapping is indeed possible and that the brain is not a featureless jungle. Note the general layout of the brain: the vigilant guardhouse of the brain stem surmounted by the halls of drive and emotion which lie under the great roof of the cerebral cortex. These

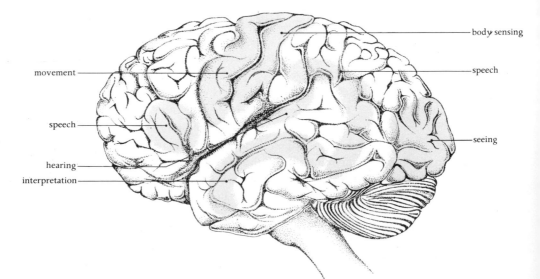

Some of the functions mapped with most confidence in the left side of the human brain. (Adapted from a diagram of Penfield)

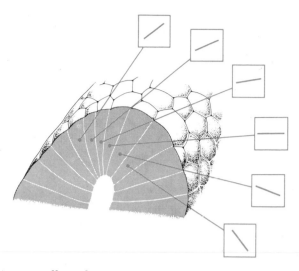

Extremely detailed mapping of a small part of the visual cortex, where information arrives from the eye. Each column of brain cells is concerned with picking out lines lying in the field of view at a particular angle, as indicated in the small squares. (Adapted from a diagram of Hubel)

regions are all amply interconnected with great cables of nerve fibres. The rear parts of the roof of the brain serve most of the executive functions of the conscious mind; the front parts constitute a profound mystery to be approached with circumspection.

Within those broad divisions we shall sample some of the particular working systems of the brain that supply mental functions, including the control of movement, the incorporation of memory, seeing and the inward seeing of imagination, and (later) the precious mechanisms of language. In some cases,

Alexander Luria distinguishes three main 'blocks' of the brain: (1) the brain stem, surmounted by the thalamus, concerned with wakefulness and response to the outside world; (2) the rear part of the cerebral cortex, concerned with analysing and storing information; and (3) the front of the brain, of elusive function but probably concerned with intentions and plans.

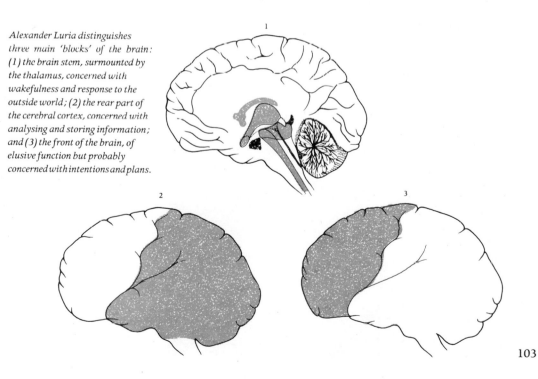

the localisation of function turns out to be amazing, going right down to individual, specialised brain cells that pick out each of the sloping lines of this letter 'V' that you now see. But in the other mental functions the brain operates in a much more versatile and baffling manner.

Movement to order

A well-defined region in the roof of the brain has detailed control of the muscles that produce movement. It is a strip about an inch wide, at the forward side of the deep fold that runs athwart the middle of the brain. Within it are big cells with long fibres; they fire off instructions to the muscles, via relays low in the brain.

At various points along this motor strip, each part of the body is represented. On the left side of the brain, controls for the right side of the body are laid out, and vice versa. That is the main pattern, but each side of the motor strip has some control over its own side of the body. Hand and mouth have big shares of the motor strip. When a patient is conscious during a brain operation, the surgeon can give electrical stimulation in the motor strip and produce definite movements: here a twisting of the foot, there an arm movement, at a third point a clamping of the jaw. Penfield and his colleagues in Montreal have mapped the motor strip in detail.

Never do patients stimulated in the motor strip have the feeling that they want to make the movement; on the contrary, they are usually rather surprised. One patient, quoted by José Delgado, tried unsuccessfully to prevent a hand-clenching movement produced by stimulation and remarked: 'I guess,

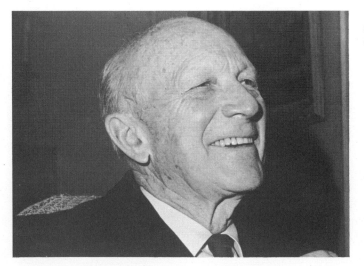

Wilder Penfield, Canadian brain surgeon and an outstanding explorer of the living human brain.

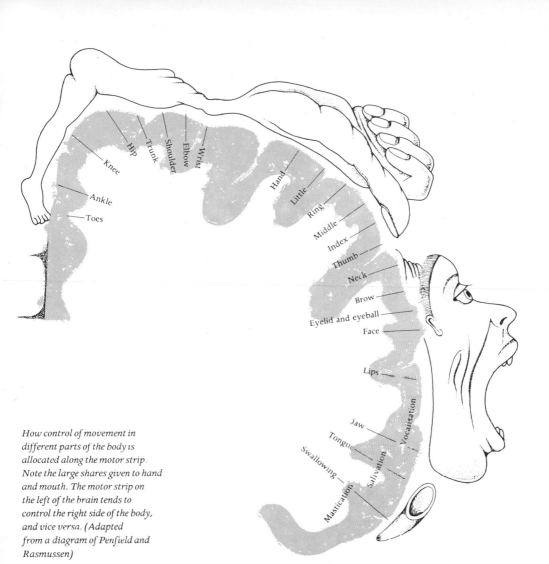

How control of movement in different parts of the body is allocated along the motor strip. Note the large shares given to hand and mouth. The motor strip on the left of the brain tends to control the right side of the body, and vice versa. (Adapted from a diagram of Penfield and Rasmussen)

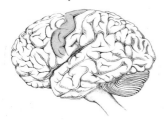

The motor strip

doctor, that your electricity is stronger than my will.' The motor strip seems to be a purely executive region of the roof of the brain. A long-held belief notwithstanding, it is certainly not a centre of will, where the administrative decision to move a limb originates.

Even in its limited, highly practical function, the motor strip is not self-sufficient. It depends for efficient operation on another strip lying parallel and just behind it on the roof of the brain – the sensory strip, also mapped by Penfield. Here the brain gathers information internally from the moving parts of the body, including precise intelligence about the position of each limb and the state of its muscles. Without this information any movement is clumsy, as it is when a leg has 'gone to sleep' or a cold face makes talking difficult. In extreme cases, when part of the sensory strip is damaged, the corresponding limb 105 may be paralysed even though the limb itself and the motor strip are in working order.

And even for an executive the motor cortex seems to be pretty low-ranking. In the late 1960s Edward Evarts, of the National Institutes of Health in Maryland, wished to confirm his belief that the motor strip issued the general command for a movement to occur – a limb to a particular position – leaving lower regions to deal with such menial questions as what forces were required in the various muscles to carry out the command. But he proved himself wrong. He trained monkeys to rattle a lever back and forth, opposed by a force which could be varied by the experimenter. Evarts then used the most modern techniques for listening to individual brain cells in the motor strip. They did not behave like aloof commanders; their activity depended on the force needed to move the lever.

Although the sensory strip and the motor strip are side by side on the surface of the brain, information does not flow directly between them. It goes by way of the so-called 'inner chamber', the thalamus, deep in the interior at the top of the brain stem. Other information and instructions flow through the same region. Any eventual explanation of how the brain produces a willed movement – a question we shall return to in Chapter 10 – will have to take the organisation of these deep-lying interconnections into account.

An impression of the connections between the roof of the brain and the deep-lying thalamus, or 'inner chamber'. Besides being a thoroughfare for information interchange, this central region may have important integrating powers. (After Nathan)

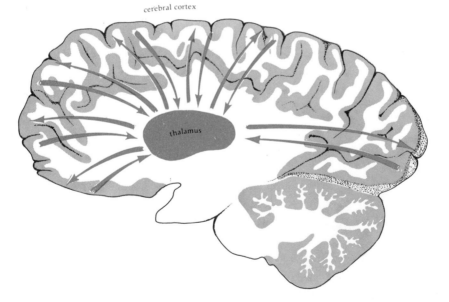

cerebral cortex

thalamus

Indeed, to think of the roof of the brain, the cerebral cortex, as the highest seat of mental function, administratively as well as anatomically, may be old-fashioned. This 'crowning glory' may be more like a huge information-processing system at the service of, rather than in charge of, the brain as a whole. The interior of the brain handles a vast amount of traffic of which we are quite unconscious. This inner system would represent, in Wilder Penfield's words, a level of integration higher than that to be found in the cerebral cortex. Penfield may be right and his point of view is a useful corrective to the customary reverence for the cerebral cortex. But it may be better to picture the brain altogether more democratically. The notion that any particular part is boss is reminiscent of the idea of the little man, or a soul, inside our heads.

Unknown universe

If you were using a heavy iron rod to thump a rock-blasting charge into place, and if you forgot first to shield the powder with sand, so that the resulting explosion drove the rod through your cheek and out through the top of your forehead, you might well expect to be dead. But an American foreman named Phineas Gage walked in to see the surgeon an hour after precisely such an accident. He went around for twenty years showing off the four foot rod.

The accident occurred in 1848 and the medical men of the time were amazed. The front of Gage's brain was largely destroyed. He continued to earn a living and he had suffered no

The skull of Phineas Gage, showing the holes through which the iron tamping bar (below) was driven by an explosion. Gage survived, but the damage he suffered in the front of his brain affected his character.

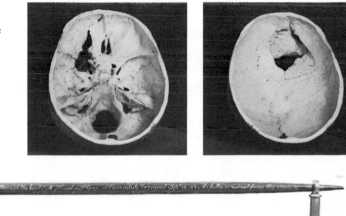

ill-effects in his memory, nor in his powers of thought. But people who knew him said he was no longer the same man. His character had changed. The formerly mild-spoken, efficient man was now foul-mouthed, impatient, obstinate, and forever making plans and then abandoning them. A doctor who studied Gage reported a disturbance of 'the balance between intellectual and animal traits'.

A century later surgeons were deliberately changing the personalities of their patients by interfering with the front of the brain, otherwise known as the frontal lobes. Egas Moniz, a psychiatrist of Lisbon, started the fashion for 'frontal lobotomies' as a treatment for mental illness, after hearing how Carlyle Jacobsen at Yale had made a mentally disturbed chimpanzee relaxed and cheerful by removing a large part of the front of her brain. In the 1940s, surgeons less cautious than Moniz, particularly in the United States, were carrying out thousands of such operations each year, while Moniz himself was given a Nobel prize.

As a relief of the terrible suffering of severe mental illness, the operation usually worked. But many patients were dehumanised. They were often reduced to clever animals with no determination, careless of the results of their actions, apathetic. A lawyer who asked for a lobotomy was worried because he got violently drunk from time to time. Afterwards he still got violently drunk – but he no longer worried about it. Subsequent refinements in the operation have maximised the relief of anxiety and minimised other effects on personality. The modern procedure cuts only the connections between the frontal lobes and the hypothalamus, deep in the brain, which contains sites for control of drive and emotion. Happily, though, psychiatrists and surgeons have now largely abandoned frontal lobotomy in favour of treatment with drugs.

Despite all these hints that the front of the brain has an important bearing upon personality and foresight, it remains the most mysterious part of the human mechanism. The frontal lobes make up a quarter of the entire roof of the brain and, at least in an approximate sense, they provide spare capacity not tied to specific tasks of sensing, learning or acting. This unknown universe of billions of brain cells, lying just behind your forehead, has functions only a few of which can be guessed.

Compared with the rest of the brain, the frontal lobes are relatively larger in humans than in other animals. They are the latest product of evolution and the tall human forehead is required to accommodate them. For a long time, therefore, the bump feelers were not alone in imagining that the front of the brain housed the human wits, skills and creative faculties. We now know that is not so. But, if the frontal lobes play neither a routine nor an intellectual function, what on earth are they

for?

Even their implication in personality and planning has been challenged. Wilder Penfield once operated on the slightly damaged frontal lobes of an epileptic. Before the operation, the young patient was highly irresponsible. Afterwards, when less of his frontal brain remained intact, his performance in IQ tests was noticeably higher, and his social conduct became normal. Donald Hebb, working with Penfield, commented that the patient had 'more initiative and planned foresight than many persons with frontal lobes intact'. Nevertheless, as we shall see when we return (in Chapter 10) to gaze again into this strange human firmament and listen to current opinions, the weight of the evidence is that our front brain is indeed very precious to us.

The minute-man

The front of the brain is a great, palpable region whose functions remain obscure. By contrast, among the best-known functions of the brain there is one for which no special region can be found – namely, the storage of memory. No aspect of the workings of the brain is more important or more fascinating than memory, and none is more chastening for anyone seeking to describe the machinery of mind, the greatest difficulty being the discovery that it seems to be stored nowhere in particular. Karl Lashley, a famous American experimenter, spent most of his career trying unsuccessfully to find the places in the brain where memory resided.

Lashley's method was tough but straightforward. He attacked the brains of living animals, cutting connections, carving out large portions of the brains. He did terrible things to the animals, but nothing that left them alive robbed them of previously established memory. For example, he taught rats to perform a task depending on sight and then deleted ever larger segments from the region of the brain concerned with vision. He found that as long as he left a small portion – any portion – of this visual cortex intact the animals could still carry out the tasks, and even learn new tasks. Lashley was eventually moved to say that learning ought to be impossible! The more realistic interpretation of his results is that learning occurs almost anywhere and everywhere.

Although the stores for long-term memory must be widely diffused through the brain, at least part of the machinery for implanting it is not. It depends upon a region of the brain called the hippocampus, just inside the temple, under the eaves of the temporal lobe. This is one of the few positive pieces of information so far available about memory mecha-

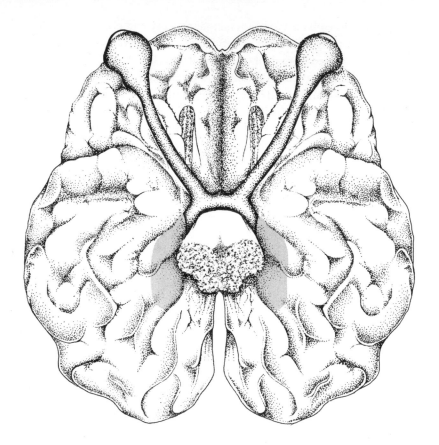

nisms in the brain. Once again it comes from the personal tragedies of brain damage in humans. One of the strangest cases is that of a man who has virtually no capacity for establishing new long-term memories. Known in the medical literature as 'HM', he is an American who in 1953, at the age of 27, underwent a brain operation for severe epilepsy.

View of the human brain from below, showing regions required for implanting memory. They lie on the underside of the temporal lobe. If they are destroyed on both sides of the head, the person can remember very little for more than a few minutes.

The surgeon removed parts of the temporal lobes, in the process greatly damaging the memory-implanting apparatus on both sides of the head. In the light of what happened in this and similar cases in the same American hospital, no such operation would now be performed. Since 1953, HM has lived from minute to minute. He can remember his life more or less up to the time of his operation, but nothing since, except for a few minutes at a stretch.

HM is intelligent, well behaved and normal to the casual observer. He does well in tests of short-term memory. If he encounters someone with whom he spent the day before he has no recollection of having met them. He will read the same copy of a magazine repeatedly, with evident fresh interest each time. He will assemble the same jigsaw puzzle over again with no sign of improvement or familiarity. His family has moved since

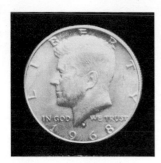

the operation and he is vague about where he now lives. Brenda Milner of the Montreal Neurological Institute, who has followed HM's case closely, quotes him as saying to her rather anxiously one day: 'Right now, I'm wondering. Have I done or said anything amiss? You see, at this moment everything looks clear to me, but what happened just before? That's what worries me. It's like waking from a dream; I just don't remember.'

Very rarely, HM surprises those who know him. In 1968 he recognised President Kennedy's head on a half-dollar coin, named him and said that he had been assassinated.

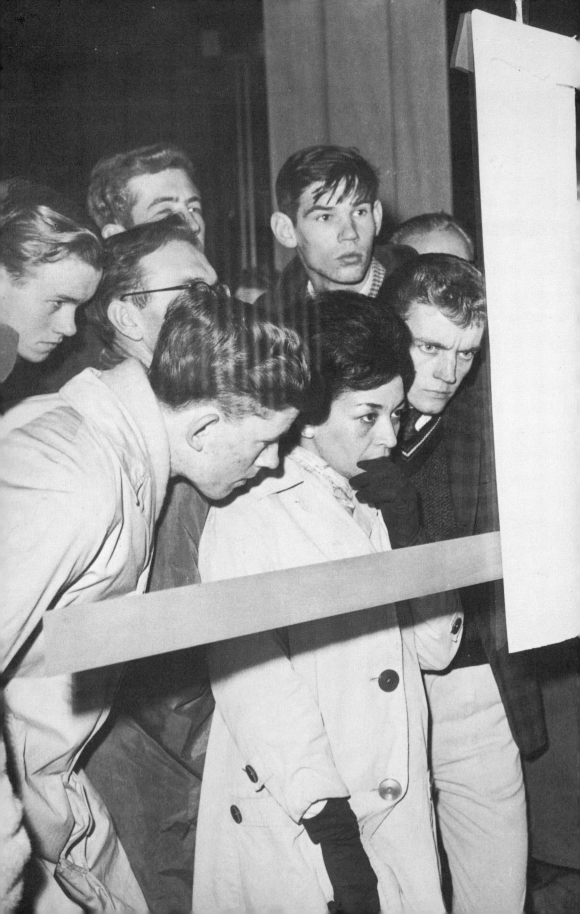

7

Store of a Lifetime

*No mechanism of the mind is more important or more perplex-
ing than memory and so this chapter ranges widely through
the subject. We encounter a Muscovite memory man, the
scientists who believe that knowledge can be injected like a drug
and some theoretical ideas about how memory may work.*

News of the Dallas shooting.

What were you doing when you heard the news that President
John Kennedy was shot?

The tragedy at Dallas occurred as long ago as 1963, yet the
chances are that your recollection is peculiarly vivid. You may
remember where you had been, what you were doing, whom
you were with, perhaps even which foot was bearing your
weight. The question is strangely evocative, not only in the
United States but around the world, in Europe, Japan, India
and elsewhere. Even HM, the man who almost completely lost
his mechanism of memory ten years previously, is aware of
this event. Each of us is haunted by powerful private memories
of danger and denouement, but here is one that a substantial
part of the world's population has in common.

Such a phenomenon demands explanation. Robert Livingston of the University of California, San Diego, cites it as a
remarkable example of a commonplace mechanism. At critical
moments, the brains of humans and animals stamp a great deal
of what is happening into the memory. Livingston believes
that this 'now print' mechanism, as he calls it, makes good
biological sense. If an animal is ambushed by a predator, and
escapes, it must learn to avoid making the same mistake again.
But what was the mistake? In the heat of the moment the brain
cannot analyse all the circumstances, so a mechanism that
remembers every clue, however trivial, for subsequent examination, gives advantages of survival.

But the registering of so much detail is a rare occurrence.
Selectivity is cardinal to the normal operation of memory and
without it our minds would drown in an excess of information.
Even as the raw information comes into our heads from the outside world, it is being evaluated and analysed by the brain. 113

Most of it is probably forgotten, but that which is remembered goes into storage through a series of stages.

If someone tells you his telephone number, for no more than about half a second you know many things: how his lips moved, what his eyes were doing, and so on. This is the fleeting moment of 'iconic', portrait-like memory. All that sort of information is promptly allowed to decay, because you are concentrating on the telephone number. You may look for patterns – is it, for example, an historic date (1945?) or an arithmetical code (6834? 68 ÷ 2 = 34). If you find no such trick you just have to rehearse the number to yourself. And if, while you are doing that, somebody comes in and shouts 'Fire!' the commotion will almost certainly drive your short-term memory of the number right out of your head.

Provided you are left reasonably undistracted, the telephone number will plant itself in your long-term memory. It takes about an hour for the implantation to occur properly, and drugs or electric shock or a knock on the head during that period can prevent it. Thereafter it can remain indefinitely in your long-term memory, though it will tend to be lost in an excess of similar information – other telephone numbers, in this case.

Mistakes of memory are also revealing. When information is still in the short-term memory, the errors are likely to involve similarity of sounds or form; the place name Lord's Bridge may come back as Longbridge. But the next day, when the name is in the long-term memory, it may be recalled as King's Bridge; the error is likely to be a confusion of similar meanings. This change implies a different kind of filing system, like a changeover in a library from classifying books by author to classifying them by subject.

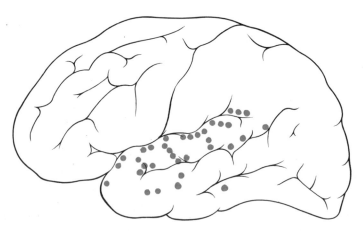

Points in the temporal lobes where electrical stimulation produced psychic responses – sights or sounds of an illusory kind. (After Penfield)

Particular memories can be evoked by electrical stimulation of the brain during operations and Wilder Penfield gives uncanny narratives of what happens in such circumstances. Stimulation of most sectors of the brain has no 'psychical' effect. But when the electrode touches the temporal lobes at the side of the brain, which Penfield calls the 'interpretive cortex', it can evoke responses like random flashbacks into a patient's past. The following are quotations from patients in Penfield's operating theatre:

'I had a little memory – a scene from a play. They were talking and I could see it.'

'A familiar memory – the place where I hang my coat up – where I go to work.'

'I can see Seven-Up Bottling Company.'

'Yes, Doctor! Now I can hear people laughing – my friends – in South Africa.'

'My mother is telling my brother he has got his coat on backwards. I can just hear them.'

To the patients, these flashbacks seem very vivid, and for Penfield they are evidence that the brain retains a complete and permanent record of the stream of consciousness. Other experts are sceptical. For example, Ulric Neisser of Cornell University, while not denying that possibly the brain may keep a complete record of an individual's lifelong experience, considers that Penfield's evidence for it is insufficient. He argues that, even if these 'flashbacks' are not dreamlike fantasies, the fact that some events are remembered is not proof that nothing is forgotten.

Penfield tells of another strange effect, this time involving speech and the recall of words, which can be produced by

Points in the brain where electrical stimulation left the patients able to speak but unable to name objects shown to them. (After Penfield)

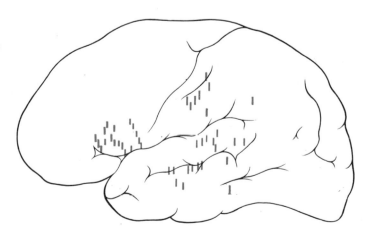

stimulation in the speech areas lying on the left side of the head in right-handed patients. This effect is not confined to the temporal lobe. Stimulation at certain points leaves the patient able to speak but unable to name particular objects: 'Oh, I know what it is. That is what you put in your shoe.' In this case when the electric current was removed the patient immediately said 'foot'.

A prodigious memory

For those of us who tend to uncertainty about even our own telephone number, there is poignancy in the story of the Russian memory man, 'S', who would write down what he had learned and then burn the paper, in a desperate but futile effort to forget. The story had a happier sequel, when S discovered how to forget by willpower. But he continued, like other prodigies, to pay a high price for his abnormality. When feats of the mind become extraordinary enough for audiences to pay to observe them, psychologists, too, may take notice. Find out how the calculating prodigy or memory man does his tricks, and there may be clues to the workings of more ordinary minds. The case of S makes a striking contrast with HM, the American brain patient who can remember almost nothing.

S was a Jewish journalist turned memory man. He was the subject of the most thorough investigation so far of any mental performer. He could memorise an elaborate table of numbers, or poetry in a language unknown to him, or a string of nonsense words, or a complicated mathematical formula, and recall them many years later. Alexander Luria, the eminent psychologist whom we met before, studied S on and off for nearly thirty years, from the day when he came into Luria's laboratory and asked to have his memory tested. In a charming little book, Luria exposes *The Mind of a Mnemonist* and remarks that it would be hard to say which was more real for S: 'the world of imagination in which he lived, or the world of reality in which he was but a temporary guest.'

A description, though hardly an adequate explanation, can be given of how S's memory worked. He would make complicated but very durable pictures in his mind. To memorise a long series of words, he would take a mental walk along Gorky Street and put an image for each word at a house or in a shop window. At first it was complicated: if the word *America* came up, he had to stretch a rope from Gorky Street across the Atlantic; later, as a professional memory man, he learned to economise in such a case, by putting up an image of Uncle Sam among the other objects in the street.

In other tasks, he would embed elaborate visual puns in little stories. For example, to fix one word, *smarrita*, in the midst of an Italian poem, S would picture a Jew sitting in a streetcar reciting the *Shmah Israel*, with his daughter (Rita) beside him. This faculty was related to an unusually pronounced mixing of his sensations, between the different senses, for example in perceiving sounds as coloured material. 'What a crumbly, yellow voice you have!' he remarked to one of Luria's colleagues.

S was sometimes at an advantage in everyday situations where he could exploit his extraordinary capacity for detail, or his power to form vivid mental pictures. For a time he worked as an efficiency expert. But in most respects his peculiar mind was a liability. On one occasion before a court hearing, he carefully prepared what he was going to say, while visualising the scene. When he arrived in the courtroom, it was different from what he had expected – the judge was sitting on the left instead of the right. As a result S lost his head – and his case.

Luria records a laboratory test during which S made his pulse rate increase from its normal 70 to 100, and thereafter slowed it down to 64. Afterwards S explained how he did it: first he saw himself running for a train, and then he imagined himself in bed, going to sleep. In another experiment, S made his right hand warm and his left hand cold, as measured with skin thermometers, by thinking that the one was touching a stove and the other squeezing a piece of ice. S also claimed that he felt no pain when his teeth were being drilled, because he simply imagined someone else was sitting in the chair in his stead.

S's vivid mental images conflicted with reality. He would see himself getting up and dressing, when in fact he was still lying in bed. But Luria is careful to point out that the 'he' and 'I' of S's imaginings – 'he' who is dressing while 'I' am still in bed – have little in common with the 'split personalities' with which psychiatrists are accustomed to dealing. S was above all a daydreamer who found it hard either to stick to the subject of conversation or to follow a career. He passed his life waiting for 'something grand', undefined, that was about to happen to him.

Luria is content to record S in fascinating detail, without constructing any special theories around him. Jerome Bruner of Harvard University tentatively describes S as one in whom the immediate fading of memory was defective, so that images normally lost within a second or two haunted S for hours. There was apparently also a failure to organise the memory and to draw general conclusions from particular experiences.   117

Here, as in more devastating forms of disorder, the abnormal case reminds us of mental mechanisms that we otherwise take for granted, and upon which depend our patterns of everyday life and creative human thought. Science and philosophy would not progress if, like S, we all inescapably saw an abstract concept, 'higher pressure', as a puff of steam moving upwards!

Knowledge in a test-tube?

Karl Lashley's failure to find any unique location for the memory store in the brain is amply supported by evidence from human brain injury. It is not amnesia which is surprising after brain damage; it is the frequency with which memory seems unimpaired. Each item of memory is repeated many times over, diffusely through the brain. We can also be confident that memory is not retained in the electrical activity of the brain. If an animal, having learned a task, is chilled under anaesthetic until all electrical activity in the brain ceases, on recovery he will then show that his memory of the task is unaffected. The general conclusion is that memory storage is essentially a chemical process.

Brain researchers can agree that memory involves chemical changes in the brain, but divide into warring camps about the nature of those changes. In one camp are 'the Believers' – a name that some of them apply good-humouredly to themselves. Their supposition is that memory consists of actual chemical molecules carrying learnt information, in much the same way that the chemicals of the genes embody inherited information. It is just as startling in its implications as extrasensory perception (ESP) and experimentally its status is similar. That is to say, there have been many tests but not one sufficiently 'clean' and reproducible to convince the unbelieving or even to give the Believers confidence.

The claim is that memory can be transferred from one animal to another by injection and similar means. James McConnell of the University of Michigan, for long an exponent of memory transfer, once reported an experiment in which flatworms learned by eating the remains of other, well-educated flatworms. Like other experiments of McConnell's this one attracted much interest and provoked the joke about mincing up professors and feeding them to the students; while McConnell himself speculated more seriously about synthesising knowledge in a test-tube and teaching by injection. 'Education' of a flatworm in McConnell's experiments consisted of conditioning the animal to contract in response to a light, much as Pavlov's dogs salivated in response to a bell.

118

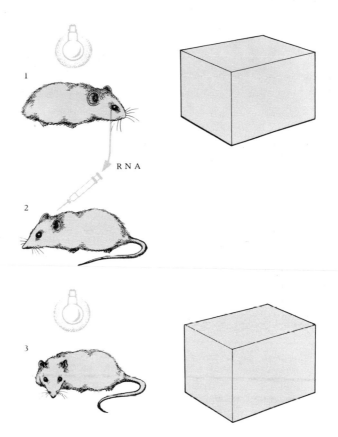

One of the more famous of the experiments in the chemical transfer of memory, done by Allan Jacobson and his colleagues. (1) Hamster learns to go into a feeding box when it sees a flashing light. (2) Chemical material (RNA) from the brain of the hamster is injected into an untrained rat. (3) The rat turns towards the feeding-box when the light flashes. Disagreement about the credibility of this and other results has divided scientists into 'believers' and 'non-believers'.

By 1965, reports were coming of memory transferred from hamsters to rats by injection. Allen Jacobson, a former member of McConnell's group, was working at the University of California, Los Angeles, when he trained hamsters to respond to a signal by entering a feeding-box. He then killed the hamsters, took a chemical, RNA, from their brains and injected it into the bloodstream of untrained rats. (RNA is ribonucleic acid, a material similar to DNA of which the genes are composed and which carries the 'written' messages of heredity.) The injected rats then showed, Jacobson said, a definite tendency to turn towards the feeding-box when the signal was given. Taken literally, the experiment meant that the chemical carried, from hamster to rat, the message 'go to the feeding-box when you see a flash of light'.

This sort of thing was too much for the non-believers, especially as it was hard to see how any of the injected material could enter the brain chemically unchanged. Yet even some sceptics have continued to investigate the alleged memory transfer. As with ESP, it is proving just as difficult to establish that transfer does not occur as to show convincingly that it does. And so long as there remains any chance that the Believers

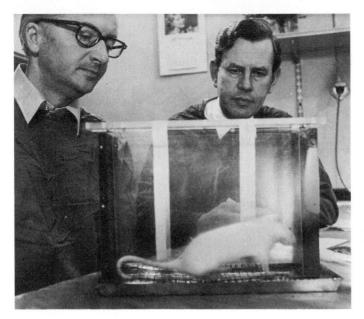

Holger Hydén (left) and Paul Lange of the University of Göteborg, Sweden, with a rat in a plastic box. From their extremely delicate analyses they have told of chemical changes occurring in the rat's brain cells when it learns to use its 'wrong' paw to reach its food. The box confines the rat in such a way as to force that action.

are right, the benefits in explanations of the brain are potentially immense. But, writing in 1970, I am guessing that they are wrong; otherwise the shape and content of this book might have to be very different.

Chemistry under the microscope

It is possible to suppose that memory is stored in specific molecules within brain cells without engaging in, or believing in, memory-transfer experiments. One of the most noted investigators of chemical changes occurring within brain cells during periods of learning is Holger Hydén. With Paul Lange, at the University of Göteborg in Sweden, he has perfected techniques which are among the technical wonders of current brain research.

Hydén and Lange deal in a most delicate kind of chemistry which is done under the microscope. They are out to discover exactly what chemical materials are made by brain cells which are involved in a learning process. They are analysing materials weighing in aggregate less than a millionth of a gramme, drawn from a mere couple of hundred brain cells in a rat. In their current work they are looking for newly-formed molecules of proteins.

They separate the various kinds of protein molecules by drawing them, with electricity, through a jelly in a very fine tube. Different molecules travel at different speeds and so separate into bands. Before its last training session, the rat has

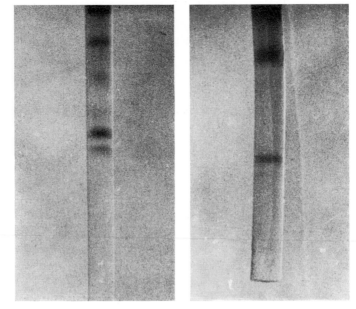

Bands of protein from brain cells of a trained rat (left) and an untrained rat (right), in the jelly used for analysis. The bands are made visible by staining. A conspicuous difference is the extra, lowermost band from the 'trained' cells. It is believed to be a modified form of the brain protein S100.

been injected with a radioactive chemical that is incorporated in newly-made protein. Proof that the material in a band was made during learning is given by measurements of radio-activity, in a small and sensitive geiger counter.

In earlier experiments, these Swedish microchemists were interested in other materials in the brain, involved in learning. The brain contains large amounts of the nucleic acid RNA. This material, which we have already encountered in Jacobsen's 'transfer' experiments, is closely involved in the manufacture of new protein. Hydén argues that RNA is exceptionally important in brain mechanisms. For a start, the RNA in the brain changes during life, both in amount and in chemical composition. In rats, it is low at birth but rises sharply in the second week of life, the period in which the animals open their eyes for the first time. The RNA content of the brain cells remains high in adult life until, with old age, it falls off again. In humans, too, the amount of RNA in the cells of the spinal cord falls off noticeably in old age.

Such is the overall trend during life, but RNA content also varies in the short term. Sustained activity in the brain, as when an animal is learning, is accompanied by an increase in the amount of RNA, and by a change in its chemical make-up. The amount of protein in the brain cells also increases, suggesting that the RNA is carrying out its function of making new protein.

Hydén's first main experiments (reported 1962–5) showed these effects very strikingly. In one series of tests, right-handed 121 rats learned to use their left hands to reach their food. That meant that the chief work of learning was being done by the right-hand side of the brain. For left-handed rats, the scheme was reversed. A comparison of brain cells on the two sides of the same brain would therefore show up any differences in RNA content. It turned out that, on the 'learning' side, the RNA in the brain cells increased steadily from day to day during training, eventually doubling after nine days. The extra RNA that was being produced altered in quality during this period.

Other brain research has supported Hydén's view that RNA is closely involved in learning. For example, Victor Shashoua, in experiments at the Massachusetts Institute of Technology, attached floats under the jaws of goldfish, which turned them upside-down and lifted their heads. Three hours' hard learning was necessary for the fish to discover how to swim the right way up and level with such an encumbrance. Pronounced changes occurred in the RNA of the brains of the fish.

In 1970, Hydén and Lange reported the first identification, in the brain cells of rats, of a protein molecule made during the process of changing over hands. It was S100, a material that occurs only in the brain. Close alongside it, in the jelly used to separate the various kinds of proteins extracted from the brain, was another, unidentified protein, also made during the learning process, possibly an alternative form of S100.

Admiration is universal for the extraordinary refinement of the experiments at Göteborg, but not many experts accepted Hydén's earlier view that the protein molecules somehow embodied the memory, in coded form. One of the basic objections is that it is hard to imagine how the brain could go through all the chemical processes needed to read the code, in the time it takes you to remember your wife's maiden name. And some sceptics say that all Hydén's fine chemistry only proves that brain cells continuously manufacture protein.

Earlier work on the chemistry of learning had also suggested that protein might be involved. For example, Bernard Agranoff of the University of Michigan injected into the heads of goldfish a drug (puromycin, an antibiotic) which was known greatly to reduce the rate of protein manufacture in the brain. The effect of the drug was to erase all memory of recent experience.

In Agranoff's experiments, goldfish swim in little tanks, each with a hurdle in the middle. A light can be switched on at either end of each tank, to warn fish that it is liable to an electric shock at that end of the tank. Normally the fish learns, during a series of trials, to avoid the shock by struggling over the hurdle. But if, immediately after a training period, the

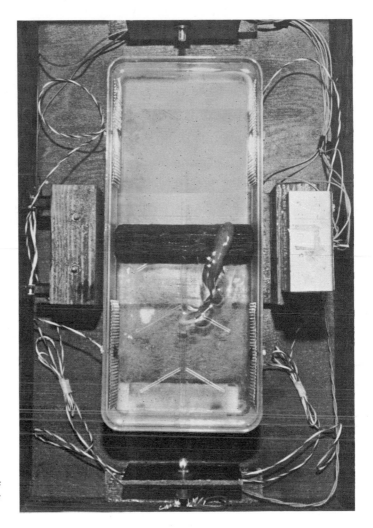

A goldfish scrambles over a hurdle in the middle of the tank to escape from the side where a small warning light is showing; otherwise it will receive an electric shock. Bernard Agranoff found that learning of this response was impeded by injections of the antibiotic puromycin into the fish's head.

drug is injected, the fish may completely forget what it had just learned, as shown by subsequent trials. If, on the other hand, the injection is postponed for an hour, its memory of the training session is quite unimpaired. In other words, vital chemical changes go on in the goldfish brain during that hour, laying down long-term memory.

This experiment and others like it, which show the erasure of learning by drugs, are as hard as Hydén's to interpret with confidence. The effect of a drug may be a simple case of temporary poisoning of the brain, as crude as a blow on the head, rather than a special intervention in the manufacture of new protein essential to memory.

Agranoff himself shares a belief with others today that all knowledge pre-exists, in a sense, in the brain. That idea is sufficiently interesting to be worth a little digression. 123

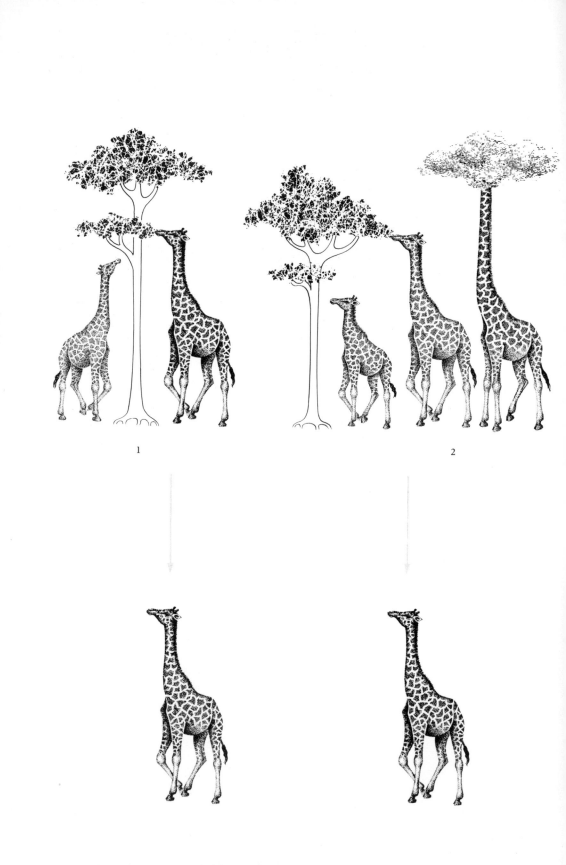

1

2

Learning or selecting?

The brain is not the only biological system capable of elaborate learning processes. Another is evolution itself, in which nature in effect learns what kinds of species can survive and which cannot. Charles Darwin's great discovery was not the fact of evolution but its mechanism – natural selection from a stock of existing plants and animals. A whole lot of species and varieties are tried; as we now know, mutations or misprints in the code of genetic instructions passed on from parent to offspring create a continuous source of experimental plants and animals. Most of them are a failure, because of internal defects or because they do not thrive in their environment. But some are selected for survival, and this process, operating over many millions of years, has produced the excellent, viable species that we know today.

A biological learning process of yet another type occurs when a man catches a disease – measles let us say. It lays him low, but his body fights and eventually overcomes the disease; thereafter, he is very unlikely to be troubled by measles again, even if he is exposed to infection. His body has learned to recognise and to combat measles, by means of specific anti bodies which attack the measles virus. The same mechanism of the immune response operates against other infectious diseases, against incipient cancer, against inert materials in cases of allergy, and against alien tissue in heart and kidney transplants.

Indeed, so vast is the range of natural or man-made materials, the antigens, with which antibodies have to deal, that it seemed self-evident that the body's defence mechanism must learn, from the antigens themselves, how to make the appropriate antibodies. But research in the mid-1960s showed this 'self-evident' theory to be wrong. Improbable as it may seem, the defence mechanism already 'knows', in principle, how to combat any one of the millions of possible antigens with an effective antibody. It now seems that what happens is that the antigen stimulates the mass-production of cells containing the most appropriate antibody. In other words, as with evolution, there is selection from pre-existing material, rather than *ad hoc* invention of new material.

This surprising discovery has prompted a German medical researcher, Niels Jerne of Frankfurt, to ask whether the same sort of selective process might not operate in mental learning. That is not a novel idea, though it stands in contrast with recent belief in the 'clean slate' of the human mind. Twenty-three centuries ago, Socrates taught that all ideas are already present

According to an old-fashioned idea of evolution (1), the giraffe grew a long neck by striving to reach high branches. Darwin discovered the correct explanation (2): nature experiments with many varieties of animals and those which have some advantage tend to survive by natural selection. A similar choice of explanations is available for learning. We may either change the structure of the brain when we learn (equivalent to 1) or select a pre-existing structure which fits what we learn (equivalent to 2).

125

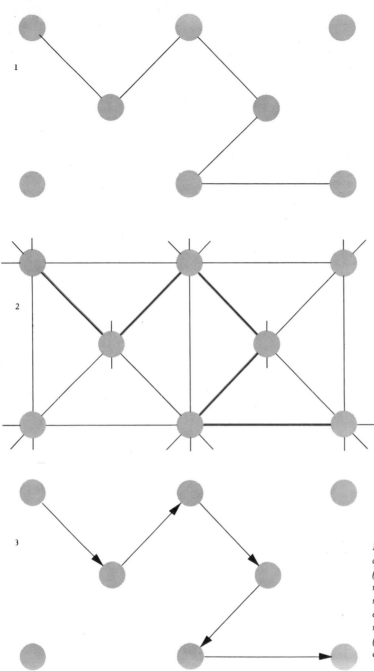

If the uppermost pattern of connections between brain cells (here shown symbolically) represents a certain experience it might be registered in the brain either by selection of one of a multitude of pre-existing pathways (middle) or by growing new connections (bottom).

in the brain, otherwise we could not recognise them when they came from outside; learning, on this view, is a matter of being 'reminded' of something that, in principle, we already know. In Jerne's view, the time is ripe to revive this theory, nowadays paraphrased in terms of the latent possibilities in the genes and of pre-existing nerve pathways in the brain which can be selected and reinforced as a result of learning.

The incident of the madeleine

Marcel Proust told of the power of a small trigger to release a great flood of recollections – one of the features of human memory that experimenters and theorists would like to explain. In his novel *Du Côté de Chez Swann*, which is known to be largely autobiographical, Proust has his narrator forgetful of most of the details of his childhood – until one day his mother gives him tea and cakes.

And suddenly the memory comes back to me. This taste was the taste of the little bit of madeleine cake, on Sunday mornings at Combray, when I went to say good morning to my aunt Léonie in her room; she would always give me a bit of it when she had dunked it in her tea or hot lime drink. Seeing the little cake reminded me of nothing; it was the tasting of it. I had probably seen so many of them since in shop-windows without eating them, that the image of the cake had let go of the memory of Combray and linked up with other more recent memories; perhaps no memory remained attached to such long-abandoned souvenirs; perhaps shapes of things – like the pastry scallop-shell, so plumply sensual inside its severely pleated case – dissolve or lie dormant so long that they go beyond the power of conscious recall. But when nothing is left of one's past, when people have died, when things have crumbled away, these two can outlast them – more faithful, persistent and unsubstantial – the sense of smell and the sense of taste. They stay on, like souls, to be recalled, to wait, to hope among the ruins of all the rest, and to carry unfaltering in their minute droplets the vast edifice of memory.

And as soon as I had recognised the taste of the bit of cake dipped in lime tea that my aunt used to give me, . . . straightaway, like the backdrop on a stage, the large, old house facing the street appeared to me, seen from the back garden where my parents had their own cottage. And with the house I saw the town, the Square where I was sent to play before lunch, the streets where I often ran errands, the good ways to go in the fine weather. And just like the Japanese game where you soak little bits of paper in a bowl of water, and watch them unfold, take shape and colour and grow into flowers, houses, and recognisable people, so now all the flowers in our garden, the waterlilies of the Vivonne, the good village folk and their cottages, the church, the whole of Combray and the country round, everything which has shape and solidity, town and gardens, all came out of my cup of tea.

The ability of the brain to store vast amounts of information diffusely through its tissues is remarkable enough, but surely even more astonishing is its power instantly to recall that information. The mechanism for fishing at random for facts breaks down too often to be consistently impressive. More remarkable is the power of normal conversation. The appropriate words flow with seeming effortlessness as human beings confer or gossip, even though each word or cliché has to be rediscovered in turn in the vast cupboard of vocabulary.

The recent invention of the photographic process called holography gives hope to some brain researchers that it may after all be possible to explain the nature and power of memory. A word of warning is appropriate here about the habit of brain theorists always to seize the latest analogy from technology. If it were not so forgivable, in view of the difficulties of understanding the brain, it would be ridiculous: the brain has been, by turns, a cooling system, a valve, a telephone switchboard and a computer, in step with advances in engineering. But it must be admitted that holography revives the spirits of

A magnified portion of a hologram, produced by photography with laser light, showing the strange pattern in which the visual information is encoded. The hologram may be a good analogy for the way the brain stores information.

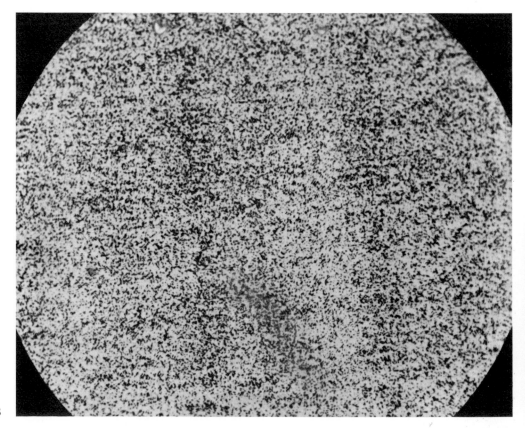

twentieth-century brain research, after Lashley's depressing failure to discover any unique site for memory. At least holography shows memory-like characteristics.

In holography, one photographs an object without using a lens but exploiting the extremely regular light waves of a laser beam. The resulting photograph, or hologram, is a very strange pattern of lines or spots, bearing no apparent relation to the object. But if, now, the hologram is viewed by the same laser light, the object reappears. Although it is tempting to linger here, among the principles and technical applications of holography, we need only note some particular features.

First, the hologram is an encoded version of the picture. Secondly (and this is where the brain experts sit up) if you develop a hologram on a glass plate, and then smash it with a hammer, you can pick up any piece, view it by laser light, and see the whole picture; it has lost some quality but it is complete. The picture is diffused through the hologram rather as an item of memory is diffused through the brain. This little test also hints at another feature of holography and of memory – the way a scrap of information can trigger the release of a lot of information, even if hazily.

From a hologram, the original scene can be reconstructed (below, right). But it is not necessary to have the whole hologram to recover the scene; a small piece will produce a degraded but recognisable picture of the whole scene (below).

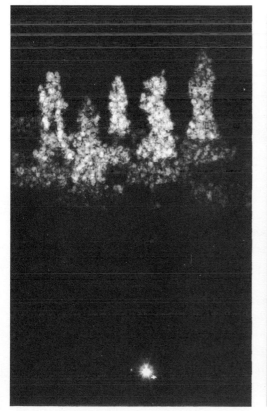
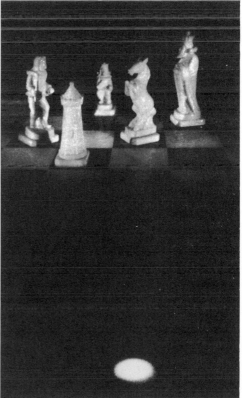

In the late 1960s there were some attempts to adapt the ideas of holography more or less directly to theories of memory and recall. One of those in the forefront of such efforts was Christopher Longuet-Higgins at the University of Edinburgh. But by 1969 he had second thoughts. It was better to take the example of a distributed memory system, like holography, but to look at it in a more general way. He and his colleagues arrived at a possible mechanism for diffuse memory storage in a mass of brain cells, which retained the virtues of holography but allowed for denser packing of information.

In this purely theoretical mechanism, a brain can hold a great deal of information, all intermixed, and an unlimited portion – but only the relevant portion – can be released by a particular combination of incoming signals. The same components of the brain can play many different roles, on different occasions. The idea is made much plainer with this diagram than

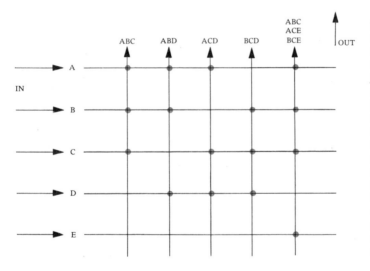

The Edinburgh theorists' version of memory storage in the networks of brain cells. Memory is represented by the connection points (the spots). A particular combination of incoming signals (from left) produces an output signal only in a vertical line fully matched to that combination. One combination of incoming signals can produce more than one output signal; conversely, the same output signal can be produced by different incoming combinations. Given millions of such links, as in each small part of the brain, the capacity for information is immense.

with words. Its essential feature is that each possible pattern of incoming signals releases a unique pattern of outgoing signals, dependent upon which of the many possible connections in the brain are effective connections.

Longuet-Higgins testifies that the mathematics allows only quite a narrow range of possibilities for brain mechanisms with a distributed memory system, which makes him confident that the brain may very well work just like this. He is sustained in this view by the fact that a young fellow-countryman arrived independently at much the same theory by a different route and fitted it to a known system of brain cells (see page 150).

There are good reasons for thinking that human beings may indeed be on the brink of discovering how their memory works. A combination of new chemical and electrical techniques allows investigators to follow in detail what goes on in the brain, aided by strong hints from mathematics about what mechanisms are likely to supply the immense power of memory storage and recall with which we are all familiar.

The wide range of current opinions about memory are a mark of continuing ignorance. The notions that memory can be transferred by injection or, less provocatively, that it resides in particular chemical molecules within cells, are hard to match with our more general information about how the brain works. Less incompatible is the Socratic proposition of Niels Jerne, which some other brain researchers also find attractive, that all possible information is already latent in our heads. An important school of thought contests the very notion of memory as a permanent store of items; instead, it emphasises a constructive process of using past experiences afresh.

The dominant hypothesis in present-day brain research, about how memory is implanted, is that the chemical change involved in learning is essentially a durable change in the connections between brain cells. Donald Hebb of McGill University stated the idea in 1949 as 'a neurophysiological postulate', as follows. When cell A repeatedly or persistently takes part in firing cell B, he said, 'Some growth process or metabolic change takes place in one or both cells such that A's efficiency, as one of the cells firing B, is increased'. In pursuit of this idea, which may well be the key to understanding how the human brain works, we should look more closely at what is known about brain cells and the connections between them.

It turns out, as we shall see, that in one region of the brain an explanation of how the 'wiring' produces its results calls upon a mechanism of the kind envisaged by Hebb.

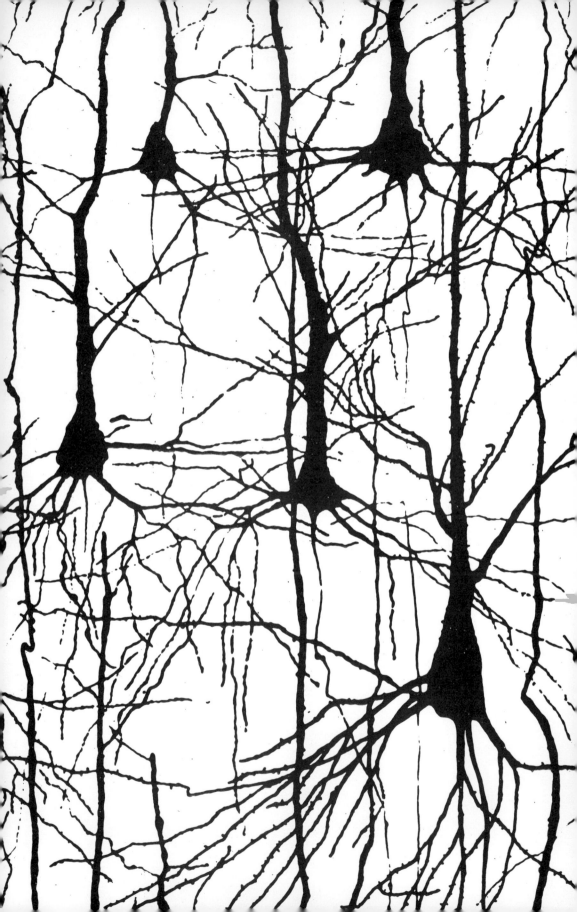

8

Minims of Mentality

Explanations of the brain must reach down to individual cells and to the connections between them. One outlying part of the brain has been well disentangled and a first account of how it works endorses the theory that the strengthening of connections between cells is the basis of memory.

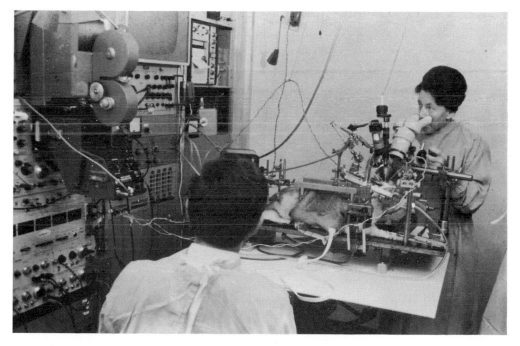

Lady Eccles (Helena Taborikova) prepares an anaesthetised cat for an exploration of the cerebellum. The work is done in a metallic cage which screens off electrical interference from the outside world.
Left: cells in an infant human brain. (Tracing by Conel)

Within a metal cubicle that seemed almost as crammed with instruments and people as a spacecraft, a party of scientists was engaged in a voyage of exploration into the brain of a cat. The animal itself lay unconscious under a blanket as a micro-electrode advanced very slowly and gently, under precise control, amid the cells of its brain. The tip of the micro-electrode, in a narrowly drawn tube of glass, was less than a thousandth of a millimetre in diameter. This very fine electric detector crept forward in steps of two thousandths of a milli-metre while all ears listened to the greatly amplified signals of

133

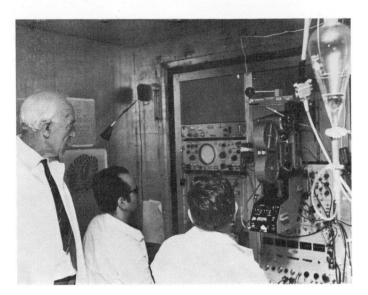

Sir John Eccles (left) with colleagues at Buffalo.

electrical activity at the tip, fed into a loudspeaker in the laboratory: silence, a few clicks, silence again.

Helena Taborikova, from Czechoslovakia, was navigator, controlling the micro-electrode with push-bottons. At last the loudspeaker began to buzz with the rapid firing of a brain cell of the type she was seeking. The young experimenters in the cubicle, men hailing from Japan, the Lebanon and the United States, quickly began using the big recording and computing panel to find out what was happening. Watching the proceedings, was Dr Taborikova's husband, Sir John Eccles from Australia, the most experienced brain explorer of all. 'Every time I come in here,' he remarked to me, 'I know there's the possibility of making an important discovery.'

Eccles gathered his young men and fine instruments from all over the world to the State University of New York, at Buffalo, to continue research that had already revealed the organisation of one part of the brain in unprecedented detail. At the age of 67, with the Nobel Prize collected years ago, with service as president of his country's Academy of Science completed, few men in Eccles' position would continue so actively in research. He does so with an enthusiasm that puts many young scientists to shame.

In the late 1950s and all through the 1960s, micro-electrodes made possible a rapid series of advances in brain research. For the first time experimenters were able to spy on individual cells of the living brain, and to see how those cells actually performed when particular events were occurring. Eccles was one of those who, with great success, drove micro-electrodes

into an ancillary part of the brain, the 'little brain', or cerebellum,

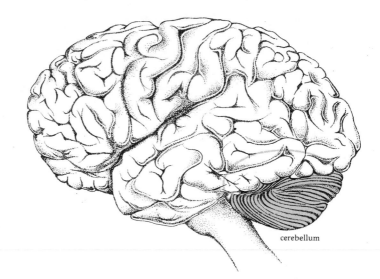

The cerebellum nestles under the roof of the brain, at the back.

which is responsible for unconscious control of complicated but routine actions like balancing and walking.

By 1970, the organisation of cells in the cerebellum was known in marvellous detail, but experiments continued, like the one I witnessed in Buffalo. It was concerned with the way internal information coming from a particular part of the body – from nerves running from the leg of the cat, to be precise – would influence an individual cell in the cerebellum. The detection of such an influence, in a type of cell that in any case fires continuously, required repeated stimulus of the nerve in question, repeated recording of the activity of the cell, and facilities to add up, average and analyse a large number of such events: hence the imposing banks of electronics and the nimble teamwork of Eccles' collaborators.

Living for kicks

If a green-fingered experimenter takes a speck of the brain or spinal cord of a very young animal and sows it in a nourishing fluid, it will grow to cover the vessel with a mass of cells. The tissue culture gives another kind of opportunity for prying into the private lives of brain cells. In their public capacity, billions of little nerve-like cells, or neurons, co-operate to make the integrated brain. In this chapter I shall call them by their official name, because they are actually outnumbered by another kind of cell in the brain. Without saying the brain is necessarily like a computer, we can allow that the neurons are comparable with the transistors and other working components of an electronic machine.

135

Cultured outside the brain, the neurons reveal their predisposition to act appropriately, somewhat unnatural though their situation is. In the microscope they show the vitality that is missing in the dead tissue which is more often examined. They can be seen taking in nourishment and growing. Materials pass to and fro within the cells. The branches whereby the neurons make connection with one another can be watched sprouting. The neurons even generate, spontaneously, the type of electric impulse that they transmit in their routine operations in the brain.

The brain contains far more neurons than there are human beings in the world. It is probably true to say that no two neurons are identical or perform exactly the same task, although there is much sharing of effort. The little neuron of the brain stands towards one end of the range of objects and phenomena out of which explanations of the mind of man have to be made. It lies in the province of the microscopist.

Not much more than 100 years ago did the biologists become certain that every tissue and organ of the human body was built of cells, visible only with a microscope, each with a life of its own. There is immense variety: bone, muscle, skin, kidney, blood – every organ requires its own special types of cells, and their development from the shapeless speck of a fertilised egg is one of the most impressive of nature's skills. Our picture of the neuron dates from 1865, when an unfinished account by young Otto Deiters of Bonn was published, two years after he had died at the age of 29.

Deiters' sketches survive the advances of a century and still give a good general impression of the neuron. Today, the electron microscope magnifies cells far more than the older optical microscope can ever do and it has greatly enlarged the knowledge both of cells in general and of neurons in particular. The advent of the micro-electrodes, for recording electrical activity in individual cells, has also speeded the investigation of neurons.

As many sufferers from nerve and brain damage know too well, adult neurons do not renew themselves. In this respect they differ from most other tissues of the body, which are continuously replicating and replacing themselves. But the fact that neurons do not replicate does not mean they are inactive or go unrepaired. On the contrary, they are continually manufacturing new protein, which is also continually lost or destroyed. Nearly all the protein of the brain is renewed every three weeks.

Apart from the neurons, there is another, even more multitudinous, class of cells in the brain, called glue because they

The first realistic picture of the neuron, drawn by Deiters a hundred years ago. It comes, not from the brain, but from the spinal cord of an ox.

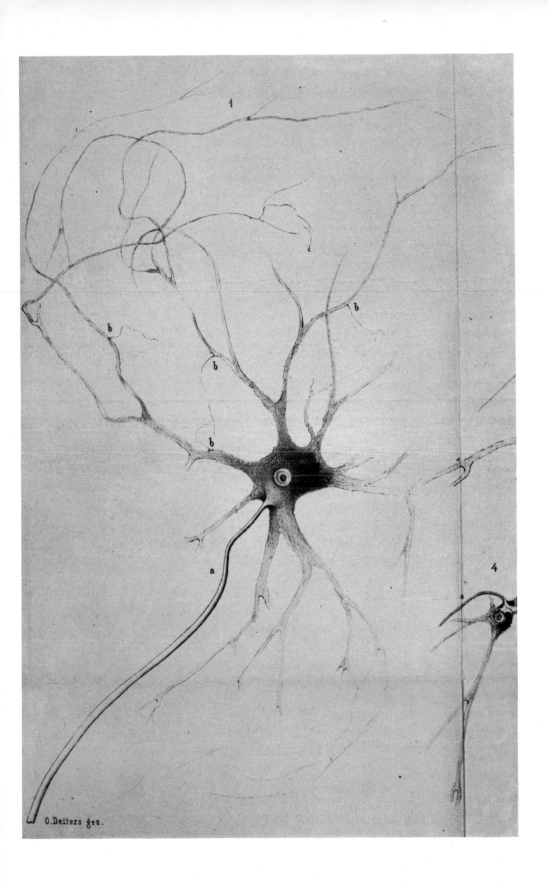

O.Deiters gez.

hold the stuff of the brain together. To make it sound more learned, the anatomists translate glue into Greek and call it glia. But, being composed of living cells, the glue is more potent than its name implies and an important task for current brain research is to discover just what other functions the glue cells serve. They certainly do not work electrically as neurons do, but it would be surprising if the neurons were not influenced by the glue cells surrounding them.

The glue cells help to insulate the neurons from one another except at the intended points of contact. They also help to service their neuron neighbours with materials from the blood and they may play a more intimate part in the lives of neurons. Whether they are also active in the thinking processes of the brain is still a matter of conjecture and controversy. Some suspect that the glue cells are involved in learning; Holger Hydén has suggested that they may send chemical instructions to the neurons for the manufacture of particular proteins.

Meanwhile, we must make the usual assumption that the prime actors in the theatre of the mind are the neurons. They vary enormously in size, shape and function, but typically they resemble a tree. There are spreading 'roots' at one end, in the

A neuron compared with a tree.

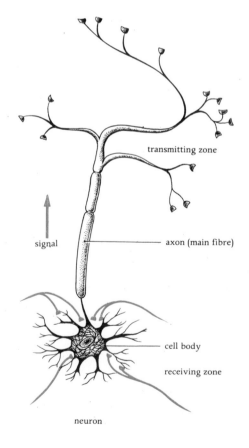

transmitting zone

signal

axon (main fibre)

cell body

receiving zone

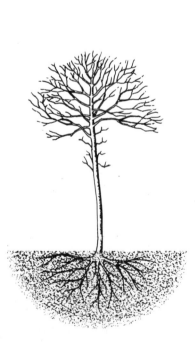

138   tree   neuron

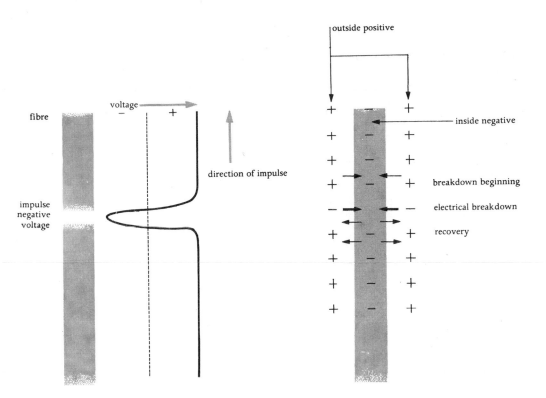

outside positive

voltage

fibre

− +

inside negative

direction of impulse

breakdown beginning

electrical breakdown

impulse
negative
voltage

recovery

How an electric impulse travels along a fibre, when a neuron fires. This information comes from studies of nerve cells outside the brain.

zone where the neuron receives signals; a 'trunk', or axon, which is the main nerve fibre; and 'branches' whereby the neuron transmits signals. In addition, the neuron has a vital blob, the cell body, which maintains the life of the neuron. The ability to fire electric signals through its trunk and branches is the most obvious special behaviour of a neuron.

In this function of the neuron as a generator of electric impulses the coat, or membrane, of the cell serves as an electric battery. It maintains a small voltage difference between the inside and the outside of the cell. When the neuron receives a 'kick' that fires it, the membrane breaks down, in the electrical sense, and the voltage on the outside momentarily drops. In fact, it overshoots, because of a streaming of charged atoms (sodium and potassium) through the membrane, and the event produces an impulse of about double the original voltage difference. The discharge at one end of a fibre triggers the same discharge in the next portion of the fibre, and so on, down to the far end.

The vote of the synapses

The artistry of the brain lies, not with the intrinsic performance of individual neurons, but in the way they interact. Each neuron connects with others, and influences their behaviour; 139

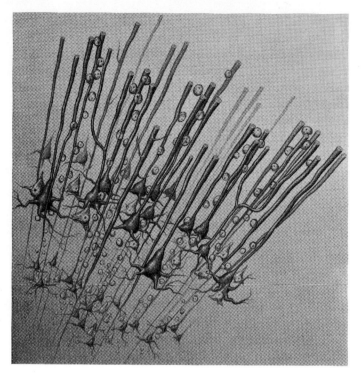

The organisation of neurons in part of the human brain, the visual cortex. The interconnected columns are about 1/120 mm apart. This new visualisation is achieved with the aid of 3-D microscopy.

that is what turns a heap of cells into a clever brain. The nerves that run through the body receive signals from, or transmit them to, the sense organs, muscles, glands and other departments of the human organism. Within the brain, neurons communicate mainly with one another. The branches of the transmitting end of the neuron are connected by sticky pads to other neurons. The junctions so formed are called synapses, from the Greek word for a contact, chosen by Sir Charles Sherrington.

Anyone who looks inside a radio, never mind a computer, can see that a fairly complicated internal circuit is needed to make the system work. The 'wiring diagram' of the neuron circuits of the brain is incomparably more complex. In the roof of the brain alone there are about 10,000 million neurons and one neuron is typically connected, by synapses, to thousands of others. Almost all the available space is filled with a felt of fine nerve fibres, appalling to anyone wanting to disentangle them and trace the circuits of the brain. The only comfort is that the circuits are not random. The neurons of the brain seem to be connected in an orderly way.

If you mash up animal brain and then spin it very fiercely in a machine called an ultracentrifuge, you can separate broken nerve endings from the rest of the brain material. Very often, attached to the nerve endings are fragments torn from other neurons, showing how sticky are the synapses that link the neurons together. Indeed this technique, developed in the early 1960s, provides a convenient way of collecting synapses for detailed study.

The synapse ranks with the neuron itself as an essential component of brain circuitry. It is across the synapse that signals are passed from one neuron to another. There is no direct electrical connection, as we have already seen in considering the mechanisms of waking, sleeping and drugs. A slot or cleft separates the nerve ending from the neuron to which it is attached. Across this cleft, about a millionth of an inch across, the signal passes in chemical form. The electric impulse arriving at the nerve ending releases a quantity of a special chemical. This material, the transmitter, is squirted into the cleft and, on crossing it, either excites or inhibits the neuron on the other side.

In the simplest case, the firing of one neuron encourages the firing of the next; the link is called an excitatory synapse. In other cases, the firing of one neuron, communicated to another through the synapse, discourages the second neuron

The vote of the synapses, represented schematically. Around a real neuron in the brain, there may be many hundreds of synapses, representing information from many parts of the brain and body.

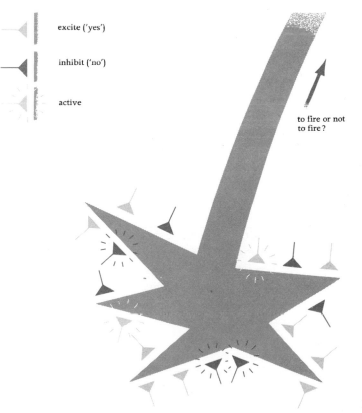

excite ('yes')

inhibit ('no')

active

to fire or not to fire?

from firing; the synapse is then inhibitory. A synapse is permanently of one or the other type. Each neuron is either always excitatory or always inhibitory in its dealings with other neurons. The choice between excitation and inhibition greatly enlarges the possible logic of brain circuits.

A neuron in action is like a delegate meeting. On a particular issue, the meeting can collectively decide 'yes' or 'no', or do nothing. 'Doing nothing', for a neuron, often means ticking over quietly, firing several times each second. At a 'yes' vote, the neuron fires much more rapidly; at a 'no' vote, its casual firing is suppressed. There are typically some hundreds of delegates at this meeting, sitting round the edge of the neuron; they are the synapses, each representing another neuron.

Some of these delegates are well known for their tendency to vote 'yes', for they are the excitatory synapses, representative of radical neurons. Others are conservatives, tending to vote 'no' at inhibitory synapses. All are under instructions from their own neurons, though, and in a particular vote many synapses may abstain. The outcome – whether the neuron in question fires more rapidly or more slowly – is democratically determined by comparing the votes of the two factions. At least, that is the story as they might tell it to children.

Closer students of neuronal politics see that it is not so simple. For a start, a conservative delegate can, in effect, vote 'yes' if the neuron represented is itself strongly suppressed, so that at the synapse the inhibitory influence is entirely removed. In similar circumstances, the radical vote becomes effectively 'no'. As in human politics, there is also a lot of activity behind the scenes. Each neuron represented at the meeting is itself subject to many influences – frequently even, by devious paths, from the very neuron whose policy is being decided.

The most important departure from the democratic ideal is that not all the delegates are equal; some have exceptional voting powers. In other words, the neuron in question is more susceptible to influence by privileged neurons connected to it, than by the others. For some brain researchers, as we have seen, the acquisition of special influence of one neuron on another across a synapse, presumably by chemical change, is the whole secret of the brain's ability to learn by experience. Like political cronies (as this theory would have it) cells that have co-operated frequently in the past are likely to go on doing so.

May I squeeze one more pip from the political analogy? The general tendency of voting in the brain is strongly conservative, in the electrical sense. Inhibition of firing is a much-favoured mode of operation. It is related only remotely to inhibition of the psychological kind, and it makes a lot of sense. As one brain researcher puts it, 'But for the inhibition you'd have an epileptic fit every time you opened your eyes'. A general role for inhibition is to blot out excessive information, retaining only what is important. It also provides an effective mode of communication – signalling by 'bursts' of silence – which saves effort in the brain at the same time as helping to avoid over-excitement.

Other necessary functions of inhibition include the avoidance of contradictions. A simple case is the well-known reflex action of the knee jerk, when the doctor taps you below the kneecap and your foot kicks up. This reflex does not involve the brain: the nerves sort it out between themselves, at the base of the spinal cord. The nerves stimulated by the tap directly excite nerves that cause the muscles on the front of the thigh to contract. But the same signals excite other nerves which in turn inhibit the nerves that control the muscles at the back of the leg, so that they do not impede the straightening of the leg.

Another general use of inhibition in the nerves is in reducing confusion in the signals to and from the brain. Signals would tend to become fuzzy if too many cells were murmuring the same message. Nature often arranges that neuron A excites neuron B which inhibits neuron A; the result is that activity in neuron A tends to be self-suppressing. It will keep quiet unless it is very strongly excited. The most constructive use of inhibition, as indicated before, is in enlarging the logical possibilities of the brain. An action can be produced, obviously, by having one cell excite another; but it can also be produced by having one cell inhibit another which was preventing the action.

Codes and passwords

An advantage of being a fish is that, if the mass of nerves linking the eye with the brain is broken, the result is not permanent blindness. The nerve fibres grow again. A disadvantage of being a fish is that human beings may anaesthetise you and cut the optic nerve on purpose, in order to see how the trick is done. For twenty years an American psychologist, Roger Sperry, made experiments on the regrowth of nerves in fishes, newts and other animals capable of regeneration. Like those of some other experimenters, Sperry's findings during this period were too spectacular, their implications too formidable, for scientific colleagues to accept. In 1963 Sperry announced results with goldfish that finally proved the point: every neuron carries signs of its identity.

143

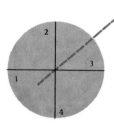

brain (tectum)

retina

Proof that each neuron has its 'password' for making the correct connections. In the experiment of Sperry and Attardi, nerves regenerating from part of the retina of the eye of a goldfish infallibly found their way to the appropriate part of the brain.

In one of his earlier experiments Sperry had shown that, if a newt's eyes were rotated in their sockets at the same time as the optic nerves were cut, the animal recovered its sight but it saw the world the wrong way up. It would dart down at a food lure passing above it. Sperry's interpretation of this and many similar results was that, somehow, each part of the eye knew exactly to which part of the brain it was supposed to be 'wired', and persisted in making the connection even after gross interference. Thus the food in the newt's view was spotted in a part of the eye which the animal's brain persisted in identifying as showing 'down', even though the eye was inverted.

The implications were formidable. It seemed unbelievable that thousands or millions of cells in eye and brain should be able to pair up again in such a precise way, after cutting. It was as if every nerve coming in from the eye had its own password which it shared only with one target cell in the brain. Unable to persuade all his critics of the credibility of such a process, Sperry could only go on and confirm its reality. In his laboratory at the California Institute of Technology, he and Domenica Attardi carried out the definitive experiment.

At the same time as they cut the optic nerves of their goldfish, they removed a part of the light-sensitive retina of the eye, whence the nerves originate. The essential point of the procedure was to leave behind, unharmed, different parts of the retina in different fish. Three weeks later they killed the fish and examined their brains, using a copper stain which made the

144

newly-formed nerve fibres stand out with a pink colour, against a black background of old fibres. What they then saw completely bore out Sperry's theory. Depending on what part of the retina remained, the new fibres ran unerringly and predictably to their own special region of the brain.

What has this experiment to do with the operation of neurons within the brain? So far, we have a picture of the brain as a vast mass of neurons, interconnected and firing according to the balance of power at the synapses. Given about ten million million synapses in the roof of the brain, it is not very hard to imagine that here is a system of immense capacity which could handle anything from swatting a fly to composing a symphony. Starting from the neuron, only the first few steps are yet possible along the road towards explaining how the system works in detail. But we can now take it for granted that the neurons are not connected randomly; the brain is not a meaningless jungle.

Nor are the patterns of firing of the neurons meaningless. They represent information in the form of a code. Some of the various kinds of codes available to the brain are known from studies in nerves outside the brain. Except when someone sticks a wire into it, the human brain has no direct awareness of the outside world. Like a manager who never leaves his office, the brain depends completely on messages coming to it from subordinates – the sense organs. These messages originate in light falling on the retina of the eye, sound entering the ear, pressure on the skin and so on. At the nerve endings in the sense organs, these influences are translated into one of the electric codes used by the nervous system. Different sense organs use different codes, and the same code can be used differently by two kinds of senses.

In the simplest code, the rate at which impulses travel along a nerve indicates the strength of the stimulus. In the nerves which register indentation of the skin of the fingertips, for example, if you double the indentation, roughly twice as many impulses will set off for the brain. Some other nerve systems simply signal the start, and perhaps the finish, of a stimulus. One of the cleverer codes varies the interval between impulses; while another registers increased intensity, not by changing the rate of the impulses, but by counting out a greater number of impulses at a fixed reporting interval, and then stopping.

A punch on the nose, or any other particular experience, is likely to stimulate many of the sensory nerves simultaneously. Comparisons and interactions of all the incoming signals provide the brain with immensely rich information from which to deduce what is happening within the body and in the surrounding world. But that kind of parallel operation of the nervous system depends on exquisite organisation, whereby the brain can tag the origin of every message.

Here enters the dazzling ability of cells to route their fibres and identify one another, as revealed in the goldfish of Sperry and Attardi. The password whereby one cell recognises another must be some kind of chemical; no one has been able to suggest any plausible alternative. It will, of course, be a completely different chemical scheme from that of the transmitter substances which carry signals between cells, once the links are established. The password is probably more akin to the process whereby the body's defences against disease recognise and attack a virus. High on the agenda of current brain research is the task of finding out exactly what the password is.

Some brain researchers have been inclined to think that individual neurons, with the elaborate chemical systems they contain, are in effect mini-brains, individually capable of great things. But most of the available evidence continues to show that the power of the brain arises from the interaction of neurons. We have encountered several mechanisms that seem to aid and influence that interaction, which we can now put in a more logical order:

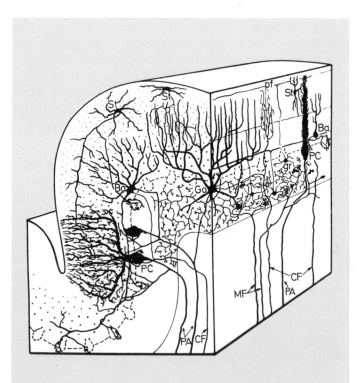

The 'wiring diagram' of the cerebellum or little brain. Left: The maze of cells in a small part of the surface of the cerebellum is sorted out by Eccles, Szentágothai and Ito. Right: A schematic diagram shows the main kinds of connections. Such groups of cells are repeated many millions of times in the cerebellum. For discussion, see pages 148–54.

passwords (chemical code) whereby neurons make the
right interconnections;

transmitters (chemical code) whereby one neuron signals
to another;

messages (electric code) whereby neurons represent information;

votes (net effect of synapses) whereby neurons influence
one another;

preferences (postulated chemical change at the synapse)
whereby, with experience, particular neurons become
more strongly connected.

Like an itinerant glue cell, we have skimmed quickly over
the neuron, noting features for which the discoverers have
already earned several Nobel prizes. In pursuit of fascinating
detail we could have spent half the book inside the electrified
coat of the neuron or swimming among the molecules of the
synaptic cleft. But, although indispensable to any material
explanation of the human mind, the neuron's contribution
may be limited.

That is Roger Sperry's view. He remarks that he has
gambled his research efforts 'on the view that the major

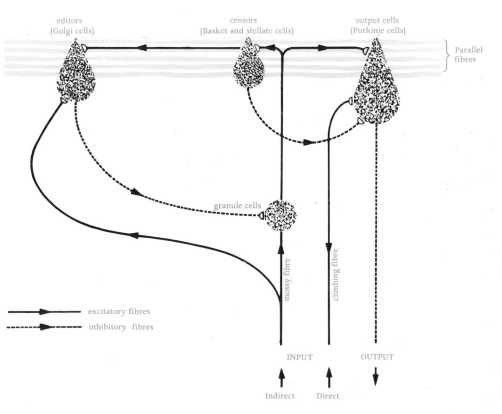

editors
(Golgi cells)

censors
(Basket and stellate cells)

output cells
(Purkinje cells)

Parallel
fibres

granule cells

mossy fibre

climbing fibre

————▶ excitatory fibres

------▶ inhibitory fibres

INPUT

OUTPUT

Indirect

Direct

mysteries in learning and memory, and in the higher functions of the brain in general, lie at . . . the level of cerebral circuit organisation'. He is sceptical of the power of a single brain cell to perceive, emote or reason; nor is he unduly impressed by growing knowledge of the activity of neurons, which he compares with 'knowing the chemical constituents of the ink and paper that have been used to print a particular message in an unknown language'.

A neuronal machine

Ideally, brain investigators would like to be able to draw the circuit diagram of the whole brain, showing how all the neurons connect with one another. So far they have approached the ideal only in one region of the brain – the cerebellum or 'little brain'. It contains an extremely large number of cells. The reason why it has been the first to yield to the investigations of Sir John Eccles, Janos Szentágothai, Masao Ito and others, is that the cerebellum is a relatively simple part of the brain, with the same pattern of neurons repeated many times, like the identical printed circuits used over and over again by computer designers.

The kind of work done in the cerebellum is made painfully clear when it is damaged. The patient may suffer from ataxia, a loss of control of movements. In a typical case, he will reach out to take another person's hand but swing his own hand wildly round it. It is a succession of errors closely similar to those of an inexpert helmsman who cannot hold the ship on course but swings her from port to starboard and back again; the essence of helmsmanship is to start checking the ship's swing *before* her head has come back on course, otherwise she will swing past it. In terms of movement in the human limbs, good control requires an orchestrated stream of signals to many muscles, telling each of them to pull or relax at just the right moment. In well-practised, purposeful movements, and in the 'instinctive' movements which help us to retain our balance, we rely primarily on the cerebellum for such control.

By 1967, Eccles, Ito and Szentágothai were able to describe the 'neuronal machine' of the cerebellum in great detail. The surface of the cerebellum consists almost completely of a vast array of nerve fibres running parallel to one another. These fibres are off-shoots of little neurons, the so-called granule cells, and provide links to the diverse other neurons of the cerebellum. The granule cells are excited by branches from 'mossy fibres' coming up from the interior of the cerebellum.

The parallel fibres sprouting from the granule cells in turn have

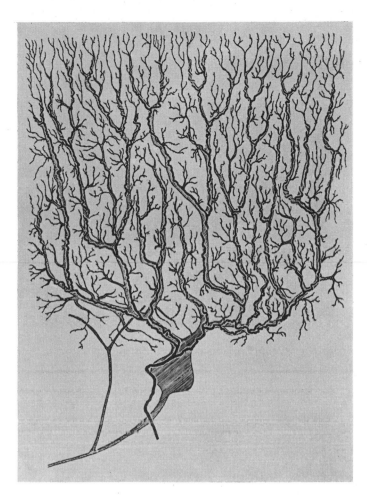

*One of the big output cells
(Purkinje cells) of the cerebellum.*

branches that 'plug in' to three other main types of cells, known technically as Purkinje cells, Golgi cells and basket (also stellate) cells. I prefer to call them, for clarity, output cells, editors and censors. All three types are inhibitory in their action on other neurons.

The big output cells are the only exit route for signals from the top of the cerebellum to the rest of the brain and the nervous system. They are excited by the parallel fibres. So, too, are the editors and the censors. The editors react upon the little granule cells that supply the parallel fibres, and thus influence the incoming signals. The censors act upon the output cells and tend to limit the outgoing signals. In a quite separate system 'climbing fibres' come up from inside the cerebellum, twist like creepers round the output cells and excite them directly.

The repetition of this pattern of cells should not be allowed to blind us to the vastness of the cerebellum. There are about 30,000 million parallel fibres in the surface of the cerebellum. 149

Each mossy fibre excites about a thousand parallel fibres (via the granule cells). Each output cell is fed by about 200,000 of the parallel fibres. Each editor cell acts on about 100,000 granule cells. Thus there is an enormous amount of excitation and inhibition going on all the time, so that one can visualise a continual tug-of-war between these two processes, the outcome of which determines what signals are eventually emitted by the output cells.

The wiring makes sense

For the first time, a wiring diagram of brain tissue was almost completely known. Admittedly, it was probably not very typical of the brain as a whole; the computer-like regularity of the cerebellum corresponded to its computer-like function. But the opportunity was there for someone to suggest precisely how the cerebellum acted. A young British theorist, David Marr of Trinity College, Cambridge, seized the opportunity and his detailed explanation, published in 1969, is regarded by the experts as very convincing. The following description of how a part of the brain actually works is a free and simplified adaptation of Marr's account.

The workings of the 3,000 million cells in the surface of the cerebellum are breathtakingly simple, once you grasp them. Inevitably they sound a little complicated at first, if only because the layout of the cerebellum is unfamiliar. So, by way of preparation, let me put the main point as concisely as possible. The output cells (Purkinje cells) of the cerebellum, which learn to operate muscles unconsciously, at first imitate conscious action. During practice, they modify their connections with the parallel fibres from the granule cells, so that they are activated whenever the circumstances make it appropriate. In essence the cerebellum is a recording machine, which memorises all the complex muscular actions involved in a particular skilled movement.

When a child first learns to eat with a spoon, he has to think about what he is doing, otherwise he is liable to forget to open his mouth, or to jab himself on the jaw. At this stage he is using the main part of the brain, including the motor strip in the roof of the brain. But the cerebellum is monitoring the whole procedure, and before very long it takes over control of the operation. The child's main brain is left free to think about graver matters, such as whether he likes rice pudding anyway. Thereafter, and for the rest of his life, he only has to make the initial decision to pick up the spoon and eat, and the cerebellum will do the rest.

What this means is that the cerebellum learns to activate its big output cells in a particular sequence, like a pianist striking the keys of his instrument. But a better analogy would be an automatic piano player which records the pianist's actions and then reproduces them as many times as required. Each output cell of the cerebellum is responsible for imitating a particular movement or correcting for it. For example, while one output cell helps to nod the head, another corrects for the effect of nodding on the sense of balance.

During the learning of a skilled movement, the output cells of the cerebellum listen to the orders going out from the motor strip to the muscles. This educational process is done via a part of the brain called the inferior olive. There, every output cell of the cerebellum has its own private informant, a reporter cell that signals to it whenever the motor strip has called for the particular action with which the output cell is concerned. That signal – a sustained burst of firing – comes to the output cell of the cerebellum by way of the climbing fibre. Its effect is to make the output cell fire rapidly, echoing the order given out by the motor strip.

But mere imitation does not teach the output cell when to become active in future. That is where the parallel fibres come in, which thread among the output cells and make very many connections with each of them. In effect, they broadcast news to the output cells about what is going on in the body as a whole. This information comes from a second eavesdropping centre, and enters via the granule cells of the cerebellum.

In our example of the child learning to use a spoon, consider an output cell responsible for opening the mouth. Immediately before it is activated, the parallel fibres are telling it, for example, that the spoon is gripped, the hand is approaching the mouth and the head is nodding forward. If the truth be told, an output cell of the cerebellum knows nothing of spoons or even arms and mouths. As far as it is concerned, some of the parallel fibres feeding it are active and others are not. Now follows a crucial step in David Marr's explanation. He adopts the idea that, if one brain cell is frequently involved in the firing of another, the synapse (or connection) between them becomes more effective. Marr applies it to the connections between the parallel fibres and the output cells, and so turns the crowd of interconnected cells into a brain-like system.

The output cell *learns* while it is active during the eavesdropping process. Any connections to it from parallel fibres that are active at the same time become more effective in future. These synapses represent the context in which the output cell is supposed to operate. With practice in a skilled movement,

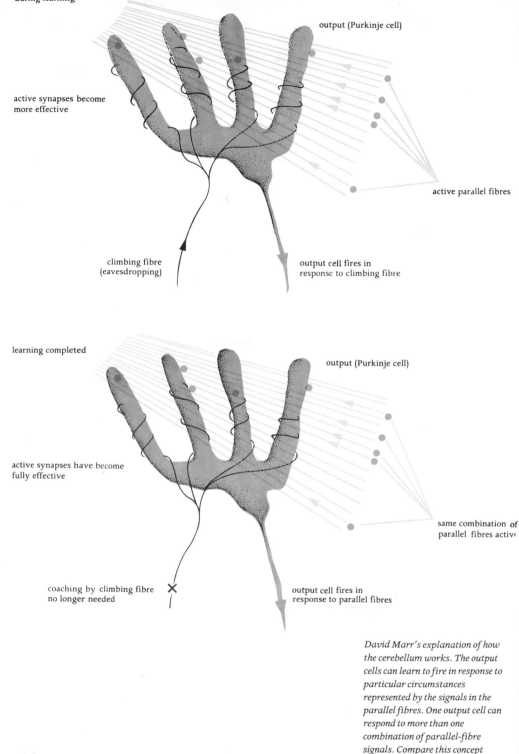

during learning

output (Purkinje cell)

active synapses become
more effective

active parallel fibres

climbing fibre
(eavesdropping)

output cell fires in
response to climbing fibre

learning completed

output (Purkinje cell)

active synapses have become
fully effective

same combination of
parallel fibres active

coaching by climbing fibre
no longer needed

output cell fires in
response to parallel fibres

*David Marr's explanation of how
the cerebellum works. The output
cells can learn to fire in response to
particular circumstances
represented by the signals in the
parallel fibres. One output cell can
respond to more than one
combination of parallel-fibre
signals. Compare this concept
with the diagram on page 130.*

these synapses eventually become so effective that the activity in the parallel fibres is sufficient to make the output cell fire rapidly.

In other words, the instruction by eavesdropping is no longer necessary. It is sufficient that a movement be started by command from the main brain. Thereafter, the fact that a movement is under way gives sufficient cues to the output cells to act in turn and to continue the movement smoothly. The skilled child, deciding that he does like rice pudding after all, fills his spoon and leaves the rest to his cerebellum.

Editors and censors

That is the essence of Marr's explanation. Its most important feature is that it easily allows the same output cell to operate in different contexts, activated in any appropriate context represented by signals in a quorum of parallel fibres. We open our mouths for other purposes than to eat. But a familiar case where the cerebellum may be operating inappropriately comes with the mother, feeding her child with a spoon, who unconsciously opens her own mouth as the spoon nears its target. The context is evidently too much like self-feeding.

Needless to say, Marr's theory of how the cerebellum works goes into a lot more detail than we have done. He tells how the cerebellum may learn to control operations that are never consciously done in the first place – a good deal of balancing, for example. And he assigns tasks to the other types of cells found in the cerebellum. Thus the editors (Golgi cells) act on the granule cells to select only the really significant information and so prevent too many parallel fibres being active simultaneously; if they were all active all the time, the output cells could not learn to recognise changing patterns of activity.

Another snag, against which nature seems to have provided a safeguard, might arise if you were too busy. There might be so much activity in the parallel fibres of the cerebellum that, by sheer accident, some quite inappropriate output cells were activated. Perhaps you would start trying to swim while riding a bicycle.

The censors (stellate and basket cells) prevent this kind of mishap. Between them, forty or so censors acting on each output cell can sample a wider range of parallel fibres than the output cell itself does. If there is too much going on all round, the censors will join forces to veto the output. As a result the output cell operates only if the signals activating it are a substantial fraction of all the activity in the area.

David Marr's theory explains the main features of the organisation of the cerebellum – the best-known, although atypical, part of the brain. It has still to be fully tested by experiment. It is probably at least roughly right, as far as it goes, though it may not do full justice to the competence of the little brain. There should be no need to apologise to the reader for having gone into some detail at this point. If the human mind could not make sense of its simplest adjunct, the cerebellum, we should have to be pessimistic indeed about understanding the rest of it.

Never the same brain twice

If David Marr's explanation of how the little brain works is even approximately correct, a lot of what we have been describing about neurons, connections and the theories of memory begins to fall into place, while some of the other ideas about how learning occurs and memory is stored begin to drop out of the picture. The fact that a process of learning by strengthening connections can be fitted so aptly to the neurons of the cerebellum gives a substantial boost to that possibility, and knocks the rival ideas.

A big question remains, about how this strengthening of the synapses is realised in practice. It is primarily a chemical question, because some permanent structural change must occur. The possibilities range from an increased sensitivity of the neuron at the 'receiving end' of a synapse, to the sprouting of new branches from the neuron at the 'giving end', to make additional synapses.

Samuel Barondes, of the University of California, San Diego, likes to relate the chemical implantation of memory to those experiments of Roger Sperry and others, on the growth or re-generation of the nervous system, showing how some kind of password or recognition signal ensured that the right links were established between particular cells. He thinks that proteins and other material formed during learning may go to make up such recognition signals between neurons, lying on the surfaces of the cells and dictating their relationships.

The evidence grows that some kind of lasting chemical change occurs in the brain whenever we experience anything or learn something, and that this is reflected in the formation of bigger or more numerous connections between neurons. By easy extension, other changes occur whenever we have an idea, as an inward experience or mode of learning.

There seems to be a philosophical watershed here, because it
is no longer possible to distinguish between mind and brain if

every mental event involves a change in the very fabric of the brain. No longer can we, for example, contrast the brain, as a kind of television receiver, with the mind as the programme that plays on it. The programme alters the receiver which alters the programme which alters . . . it really won't do. If you were watching a receiver that performed like that, would you not be inclined to say that the machine had a mind of its own?

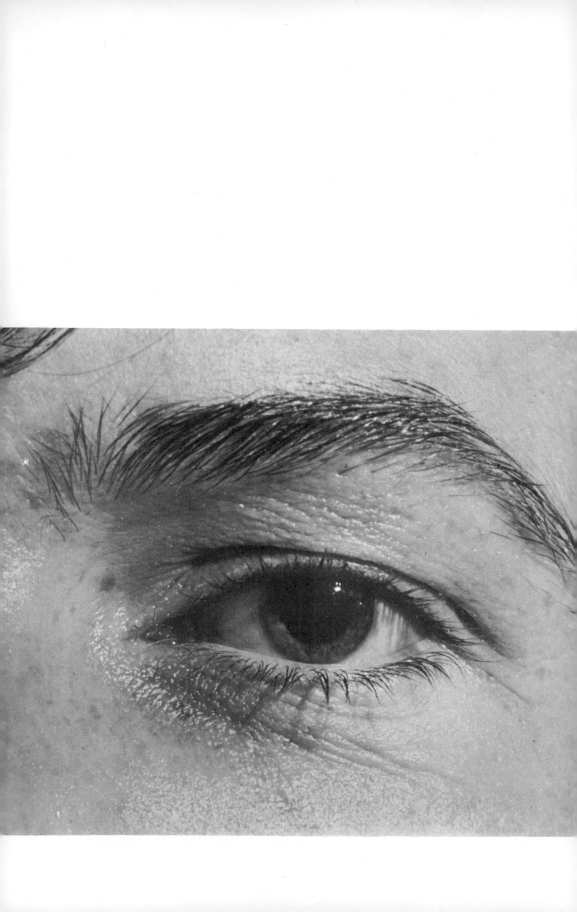

9 More than a Camera

Striking discoveries about how the brain analyses what the eyes see have come from other prying into individual brain cells. What we see is not reality but a 'model' of it and, whatever further brain mechanisms are involved, this 'model-making' serves also for visual memory and imagination.

A fire-warning detector will 'smell' smoke and sound an alarm; a guided missile will 'see' and pursue a radar echo or the hot engines of a bomber; a speed governor will 'feel' when a shaft is spinning too fast and act to restrain it. But the coy quotation marks are appropriate in all such cases, because these machines do not have minds and they do not perceive the world as human beings do. Information from our eyes, ears and other senses goes to our brains, and of some of it (by no means all) we are aware as a vivid part of our conscious experience, showing us the world we inhabit.

Conscious perception has never been easy to explain. How do nerve cells, carrying encoded information from the eye about patterns of brightness and darkness, re-create in the brain an orderly picture of the outside world, which we know to be real and which we can interpret and memorise? Seeing how René Descartes approached it three centuries ago is as good a way as any to grasp exactly what the problem is. He envisa-

The eye is an outpost of the brain, capable of preliminary analysis of the patterns of light entering it.

Below: Descartes' idea of seeing. The soul perceives an object projected by the nerves from the eye into the interior of the brain.

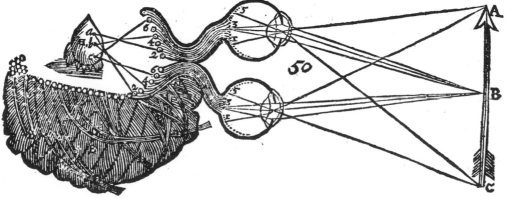

ged a television system, in which the pictures from the eye were displayed on screens deep inside the brain. The soul, sitting in the stalls, contemplated them.

In other words, understanding how the brain forms impressions of the outside world is so difficult that it seems easier to think of oneself as a little man inside the head, looking at the incoming signals. But unless you dodge the issue by ascribing divine powers to this little man, he presumably has a little man inside his head – and so on *ad infinitum*. The buck has to stop somewhere, and the aim must be to stop it in the brain tissue connected with the various senses.

We have to show that the brain tissue not only carries the coded versions of sights and sounds but also perceives them and that the conscious experience is simply part of the process of analysing the information coming in from the sense organs.

The processing of information begins in the eye itself. The ganglion cells of the retina are sensitive to bright or dark spots. For example, this ganglion may respond when its central zone is bright and the surround is dark, or vice versa.

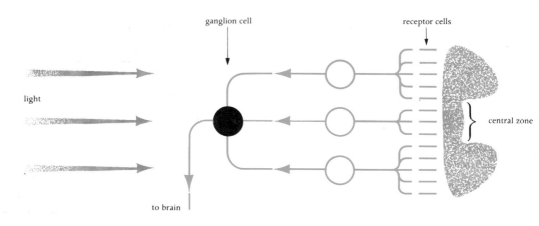

ganglion cell

receptor cells

light

to brain

central zone

That cannot yet be demonstrated to everyone's satisfaction, because we know far too little about the brain processes involved. But some mechanisms of seeing have recently emerged which give strong hints of the brain's capacity for the task.

The most impressive discoveries have been made by two men working together in Boston – David Hubel from Canada and Torsten Wiesel from Sweden. But there are historical and explanatory reasons for starting an account of seeing with the eye itself before we turn to the processes in the brain which Hubel and Wiesel have found. In any case, the eye is not a passive television camera, of the kind that Descartes supposed. It is, in effect, an exposed part of the brain, and the process of analysing what we see begins with the eye.

The lens in the front of the eye casts an upside-down image of the prevailing scene on to the retina at the back of the eye. Spread across the retina are more than 100 million light-

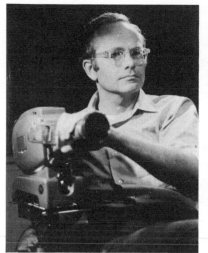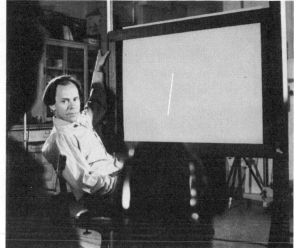

David Hubel works a projector which throws a line of light on to a screen in front of the animal's eyes, while Torsten Wiesel (right) marks the features to which a particular brain cell responds.

sensitive cells which absorb the light and fire in response to it. How those cells work, and how they detect the colours as well as the intensity of the light, is a fascinating topic in itself, though it need not now detain us. At this first stage the eye is little more than an electric camera. But the light-sensitive cells do not transmit their responses directly to the brain.

There are relay cells in the retina whose work is more brain-like. Known as ganglion cells, they gather in the signals from a number of light-sensitive cells. Each light-sensitive cell sends its signals to a number of ganglion cells, so that the fields of interest to the ganglion cells overlap to a great extent. A ganglion cell does not simply add up the signals from the light-sensitive cells in its field, it responds to particular features. In darkness, it fires slowly and spontaneously; the effect of the pattern of light and dark in its field may be to increase the rate of firing, or to suppress firing altogether.

As Stephen Kuffler of Johns Hopkins discovered twenty years ago, one type of ganglion cell fires vigorously when there is a bright spot of light in the middle of its field. Light falling towards the edge of its field will stop it firing altogether; but if the peripheral light is then turned off, the cell responds to that event with a short burst of firing. In a second type of cell the arrangement is reversed: light falling in the centre of the field suppresses the ganglion cell. Again switching off the suppressing light provokes a burst.

Antagonism between the effects of light in different parts of a ganglion cell's field means that uniform illumination has remarkably little effect on the cell. All the ganglion cells feed their signals in separate fibres along the optic nerve from the back of the eye to the brain. Each fibre carries information 159 from a particular type of ganglion cell about a particular area of the retina. A fibre coming from the centre of the retina, where vision is sharpest, represents a very small area of the retina; at the edges of the retina, many more receptor cells are lumped together under each ganglion cell.

The information about what the eye is seeing is already pre-processed. If you are staring at a plain white wall, there is relatively little excitement in the optic nerve. If you look at a small spot of light, many ganglion cells are active, and those whose fields are cut by the edge of the light spot are the most strongly affected. The organisation of the cells in the retina has provided the means of emphasising contrasts of light and shade.

Spotting the feature-spotters

The swift current of visual information flows down the optic nerve from the eye, and meets the optic nerve from the other eye where some crossing-over of nerve fibres occurs. Then it enters the brain proper to one side or the other of the brain stem. There it comes into the territory studied so revealingly by Hubel and Wiesel in their painstaking experiments with

Information travels from the eye to the back of the brain – the visual cortex – as seen from below. (After Hubel)

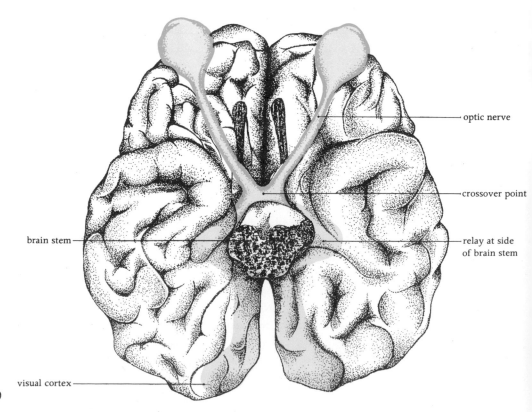

optic nerve

crossover point

brain stem

relay at side of brain stem

visual cortex

160

animals. These men have been collaborating for ten years at the Harvard Medical School, using fine-tipped micro-electrodes to pick out the activity of individual cells at work in the brains of living cats and monkeys.

The animal is anaesthetised and feels no pain, but his eyes are held open, staring unconsciously at a white screen. Through a small hole in the skull, the micro-electrode is carefully advanced into the chosen region of the brain. The experimenters listen to the loudspeaker as the micro-electrode moves forward. Eventually, after some expenditure of patience, an individual brain cell announces itself with a succession of clearly audible clicks, while the corresponding 'spikes' appear on an oscilloscope trace.

Hubel and Wiesel then move into action to find out what this cell contributes to the analysis of signals coming from the eye. They project a line of light on to the screen in front of the animal. They twist the line, move it around, alter its shape and width – all the time listening to the sounds of the single brain cell firing. Sometimes they will find out within a few minutes what sights provoke the cell to rapid firing or to silence; sometimes it may take several hours of work. Eventually they will have marked the screen to show the features of the scene that the cell specialises in spotting.

Then the micro-electrode begins its slow advances again, to find another cell. The process is repeated late into the night – as long as the experimenters and their assistants have the stamina to continue – to discover as much as possible from each animal.

Human vision almost certainly works very similarly to the monkey's vision. Cats are much more distantly related to monkeys than men are, yet the differences between a cat's brain and a monkey's brain, in the ways they handle visual information, are remarkably slight. It is not surprising, for example, that the cat is less well organised for dealing with colour information, and differently organised for judgement of distance. Where cells in the human visual system have been tested, they are similar to those found in monkeys.

Many different kinds of cells turn out to be at work in regions of the brain concerned with vision. None of the cells responds uncritically to light falling on a particular point of the retina. They all detect features of one kind or another, revealing what Hubel and Wiesel call the 'building-blocks of perception'.

At the gateways to the brain, alongside the brain stem, the processing that occurs is strongly reminiscent of the pre-processing in the retina. Here the cells are still spotting spots – 161 light or dark areas contrasting with their surroundings. But, taking in the signals from the eye, those brain cells are sharpening the information by re-emphasising the features already picked out by the retina. For example, a ganglion cell in the retina may fire when the contrast between the spot and its surroundings is not very great; the brain cells are typically much more demanding, and require very marked contrast before they will respond.

In this part of a monkey's brain, Hubel and Wiesel have glimpsed something of the mechanisms for picking out colour variations in the scene. They have found that many cells are excited by a spot of one colour in the middle of its field, but are turned off if the surround has a second colour. For example, a red spot excites a cell, a green surround inhibits it. Such a cell might fire if its owner saw a ladybird on a blue flower, but be switched off if the ladybird were sitting on a leaf.

All this processing is still at a very early stage in the analysis of the scene. As we follow the flow of signals to the back of the roof of the brain – to the visual cortex – the interconnections become more intricate. 'Stupendous complexity', is David Hubel's description of it. Yet, in the part of the cortex that first receives the information from the eyes, the overall arrangement is fairly straightforward, though perhaps surprising. Each region of the cortex corresponds to a particular region of the retina, and the regions are arranged in their proper relation one to another, across the crumpled surface of the cortex.

Here, if anywhere, would be the display screen that Descartes' soul could sit and watch. Yet the information being handled is not really picture-like – not a faithful, point-by-point reconstruction of the scene. As Hubel and Wiesel have found, the brain cells are picking out features even more rigorously than before. Just two kinds of features (bright spot and dark spot) were handled by the ganglion cells of the retina and the processors at the gateway of the brain. Each cell of the visual cortex specialises in one of very many possible features in the scene.

Nevertheless, Hubel and Wiesel have been able to sort these brain cells into broad types, which they call 'simple', 'complex', and 'hypercomplex'. 'Simple' cells respond most actively to one or other of the following kinds of features projected on to the screen in front of the animal's eyes:

a bright line at a particular location and sloping in a particular direction;
a dark bar on a light ground with particular location and slope;

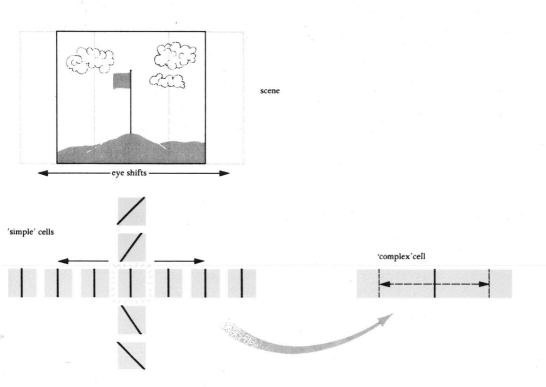

scene

eye shifts

'simple' cells

'complex' cell

Stages in the initial processing of visual information in the brain. The 'simple' cells pick out the dark vertical line in this scene, but as the eye shifts, they hand over to other cells responsive to the same line. 'Complex' cells also respond only to particular features, but they are less concerned about where exactly the features lie. They have thus taken the first step towards the idea of an object that persists independently of its precise position on the retina.

a straight edge between a light and dark area, again with particular location and slope.

Special populations of your brain cells are at this very moment having a busy time responding, for example, to the edges of this page. As your eye flicks across the page, though, different populations are taking turns to register the edge, as it comes into their precincts. If you now rotate the book slightly, clockwise or anti-clockwise, quite other populations will take over the watch on the edges, because the slopes have all changed. This degree of specialisation is impressive, but an obvious comment is that you cannot sense any of this moment-by-moment exchanging of roles that is going on in your head.

Your impression is of a book and, as far as this mental picture is concerned, it makes very little difference whether you flick your eyes around the book or keep them fairly steady. Later stages of brain processing must extract this more durable information from ever-changing activities of the 'simple' cells of the cortex. In the 'complex' cells, interspersed in the visual cortex, Hubel and Wiesel find the start of such a process of generalisation.

'Complex' cells are somewhat less fussy about exactly where features lie on the retina of the eye. They are still choosy about orientation, though. As in the case of the simple cells, rotating a line in the field of view by as little as five or ten degrees will make a 'complex' cell lose interest in it. A typical complex cell reacts to a bright line (or dash bar, or edge) of particular slope regardless of exactly where it is, and even if it is moving. Thus if you look at, say, the hands of a clock across the room, the same populations of 'complex' cells may continue to register the hands despite the fact that your eyes are wobbling and calling different 'simple' cells into play.

Perception of a constant shape has thus begun in the cells of the visual cortex that receive the pre-processed information from the eyes. Already the brain has abstracted features from the scene which persist even while the eyes move. Technically it is a small change, which can easily be explained by supposing that the 'complex' cell is triggered by any of a swarm of 'simple' cells responding to a given kind of feature. Yet the step from the 'simple' to the 'complex' cell is philosophically more profound than that. The brain has begun to shift from ever-changing responses, following the ever-changing signals in the eye, to the first idea of concrete objects lying 'somewhere out there'.

The analysis continues

Operating on the information from the 'complex' cells are further cells discovered by Hubel and Wiesel – the 'hypercomplex' cells of the visual cortex. They specialise in registering even more subtle features of the field. One example would be a cell that responds most effectively to a white block of a particular shape and size, moving across the field of view from left to right, but not from right to left.

If that makes the brain sound pretty clever, it is worth noting that Jerome Lettvin and others at the Massachusetts Institute of Technology had already, in 1959, found cells of similar properties within the eyes, not the brains, of frogs. But these 'bug detectors', as they are called, represent premature specialisation by human standards. They are so perfectly adapted to picking out only the movements of other animals – food or enemies – that a frog can starve to death surrounded by dead flies.

Hubel and Wiesel are far from being alone in their investigations of the brain cells serving sight in higher animals. After many years as a pioneer in this field of research, Horace Barlow with his colleagues at the University of California, Berkeley, recently made the first extensive study of how the cat's brain judges distances using information from both eyes. Other groups in several countries have contributed important passages to the story of vision in the brain. Otto Creutzfeldt of the

Max-Planck Institute of Psychiatry in Munich is one of those who are now confirming that what Hubel and Wiesel have found, in anaesthetised animals, holds just as well for animals that are awake. And it also turns out that there is a completely different story to be told about vision in the brain, which has nothing much to do with the feature-spotting mechanisms described here. We shall encounter this alternative method of seeing later.

By 1970, Hubel and Wiesel had begun tracing the flow of visual information, out of the areas of the cortex which first receives the signals from the eyes, into the adjacent areas where the process of seeing is carried to the next stages. In one such area in the monkey brain, many of the cells are similar to the 'complex' or 'hypercomplex' cells discovered earlier. But about half the cells are engaged in the very important task of comparing the signals from the two eyes in order to judge the distance of an object. Typically, these cells respond strongly only when the same feature (say, a white ruler) is seen in both eyes, but slightly displaced on one retina compared with the other – the way, for example, you see your knee when you are looking at your foot.

To watch in the laboratory in the Harvard Medical School as the function of a cell is teased out, by trial and error, is like the privilege of witnessing a great game between skilled players. The contest pits the brain of the experimenter against a living brain cell: is the wit of the one sufficient to nail down the intricate function of the other? The assurance with which the experiment proceeds encourages the thought that, complex though it is, the brain may not after all be a piece of engineering too clever for the brain-power of man to comprehend.

In that sense, the most impressive thing about these discoveries of Hubel and Wiesel has nothing particularly to do with vision. Rather it is the fact that every brain cell has a definite and peculiar mode of action. We can begin to see why the brain is so complex, requiring millions upon millions of cells for vision alone. Yet, on the other hand, the function of each cell is discoverable, and it makes sense. In this region of the brain, at least, the game can be played and won.

The mechanisms here studied are nevertheless still a very long way short of the full perceptual power of the brain, the power that can observe so casually: 'That's my friend John's car turning into the street and a woman is driving it too fast – oh yes, John's wife – and it's just starting to rain.' The strategy of this line of research is patiently to follow the analysis stage by stage, devoting many years' work to discover what the brain does in an instant.

While the men with micro-electrodes pursue the signals from the eye further into the brain, other researchers continue to worry about how we ultimately perceive this information. How is an unruly mass of lights and lines and surfaces transformed in your mind into a well-known face, a view of the Champs-Elysées, or the words you are reading now? In the back of the brain, Hubel and Wiesel's cells still respond to what the eye is actually seeing. In the side, at the temple, Wilder Penfield or his followers have only to touch the brain with an active electrode to evoke in the patient's mind a clear visual impression of people and places – an impression having nothing to do with what the eyes are seeing in the operating theatre.

Somewhere in between, a very important transformation occurs. The pathways of brain cells and their fibres become uncertain and, for the present, the best clues about what may be happening come from tests of the performance of the seeing mechanisms in unusual circumstances. Perception is an ancient and even now a controversial problem for philosophers and scientists. As we noted, Descartes appointed the soul as spectator; to understand how ordinary brain tissue can be the spectator remains one of the crucial steps needed for explaining the machinery of mind.

Whom then should we take for guides? Stuart Sutherland of the University of Sussex, at Brighton, has spent many years in experiments and theorising about vision. He thinks that, up till now, theories have been wholly inadequate in explaining the 'fantastic capacity' of men and animals in processing pictorial data. Sutherland recently listed some essential facts, from animal and human experiments, that any theory must satisfy which purports to explain how we recognise patterns and objects. Some particulars of a pattern have remarkably little

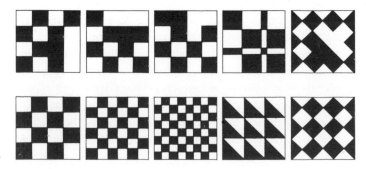

Rats can generalise about regularity and irregularity in patterns seen. In experiments at the University of Sussex, animals trained to distinguish the two patterns at the extreme left then treated the patterns alongside them as more or less equivalent.

effect on the ability of an animal or a man to recognise it. We can identify objects 'out of the corner of the eye', using a part of the retina different from what we have used before. Shown a shape with one eye, we can recognise it with the other.

Again, the size and brightness of a shape is remarkably unimportant. We are able to read a word whether it is neatly printed in a book or faintly scrawled in big letters on a wall. A cartoon outline can be almost as informative as a photograph, and it does not matter if the lines of a shape are a little ragged or crooked. Moreover, we can recognise a handwritten word even when it is crossed out with zigzag lines which greatly alter the patterns of each letter; that must mean we quickly analyse the combinations of lines in all sorts of different ways until we recognise a consistent pattern.

Yet a face in a photograph seen upside-down is very hard to recognise and certain pairs of shapes are more readily confused than others. This would-be explainer must also tell why humans can recognise a complex scene (a wedding, say) in a glance of a tenth of a second, but with little recall of detail unless there is something very inconsistent – perhaps the bride's head is missing. Given more time, we can spot lesser differences between two very similar pictures – the bride's shoes are white or black. But if no more difference than that appeared in a completely random pattern of many dots, we could never find it. We rely heavily on the organisation ('redundancy' is Sutherland's word) of the scene of real life.

Finally Sutherland points out that, although mechanisms of picture-processing in the brain are probably largely innate, a human being is able to learn about a new class of objects and to find the ways of distinguishing among them. For example, a European living in Europe finds it hard to remember the faces of individual Chinese – unfamiliar rules are needed for distinguishing them – but if he spends some time in China it becomes perfectly easy. Sutherland says that the task of explaining all these facts in detail is Herculean, but he suggests that now, for the first time, we can sketch the outlines of what goes on when we recognise a pattern. He offers his own theory, admitting that it is extremely vague.

Sutherland calls the part of the brain explored by Hubel and Wiesel the processor. It analyses the features of the scene into component lines, edges and ends. By some unknown mechanism, the output from this processor is translated into a much more abstract form, according to descriptive rules. In that form the description of the object is stored in another part of the brain. (The lower part of the temporal lobe, at the side of the brain, is the most likely place for the store.) It is in this abstract 'language' that a new picture is compared with pictures already in the memory.

'What we see,' says Sutherland, 'is not the pattern on our retina but the rule or series of hierarchical rules to which we match this pattern.' We are oblivious to normal details in a picture unless we switch in the rules that represent these details. The saying that 'you can't see the forest for the trees' seems to tell the truth about brain mechanisms. If you are examining an individual oak or fir, you are not at the same instant recognising a forest, because different rules are operating. There is plausible mathematical 'language' for describing shapes in a suitably abstract form, but no way yet of telling what 'language' the brain actually uses.

At the Applied Psychology Research Unit in Cambridge, Donald Broadbent looks at perception in the light of our shifting attention. The brain can cope only with a limited amount of information at one time. Moreover, the information may be very scanty or uncertain, when it arrives at the eye – as when we are out walking at night or in a fog. To cope with these difficulties, so that we can have some confidence in what we see, the brain has to have both a filter to cut out excess information and a procedure for using limited clues to arrive at a conclusion about what is seen. As Broadbent explains his ideas in simple language:

> Every moment your brain is gambling about which of the impressions you're getting are facts and which of those facts deserve something doing about them. Sometimes the gamble goes wrong and when that happens you make a mistake. But if the brain didn't work that way then you would never do anything right, because the environment is too complex and chancy. If you didn't have this kind of mechanism available then that complexity and chanciness would reduce you to total confusion.

Ulric Neisser of Cornell University is another respected guide to modern ideas about visual perception. Our seeing is immeasurably rich, and different investigators emphasise different elements. Thus, while Sutherland and others start with processes of recognition of essentially flat pictures or patterns, Neisser considers, among other qualities of seeing in real life, the information we extract from the texture of objects seen at various distances. In this he follows James Gibson, of the same university, who coined the phrase 'ecological optics' for dealing with the dense network of rays which come to the ever-moving eye from the surfaces of real objects.

Texture is important as a clue to distance. Without the clue of increasing density of detail we might easily misjudge the relative sizes of objects.

A simple example of the information given by the texture of objects would be that of looking at a table-cloth decorated with little flowers, from one end of the table. The pattern at the far end appears denser – more flowers per square millimetre of the retina – than at the near end. The change undoubtedly helps in forming the impression of a table-cloth receding from us. That sort of information may be very helpful if we are to judge size correctly, and not to think that a cup standing at the far end of the table is very much smaller than the one at our end.

The eye is always flickering about; the head moves; objects move. The brain adds together a great variety of impressions, at high speed, in telling us a single visual story: 'I am walking down a street and John is walking towards me tossing a ball'. For Neisser this means a process of temporary memory is at work, in which we are building up a 'model' of the scene. It is a scheme which certainly does not represent the successive impressions on the retina but extracts from each impression information that extends the 'model' or fills in details. The 'model' is what we see, and nothing else.

The discovery of a 'model' occurs very rapidly indeed, in what Neisser calls the pre-attentive process. It produces the objects that are to be 'filled in' and interpreted later. You do not see a beak, some claws and feathers and deduce that you are looking at a bird; you notice a bird. If the bird appears in the corner of your eye while you are reading in a park, you may identify it only half consciously, yet instantly. If the bird interests you (perhaps it is injured, or has a rare plumage) you .will attend to it and find out more about it. Neisser equates his pre-attentive process to the very brief 'iconic' memory, and

169

the fleeting but comprehensive experiences which are mostly forgotten.

The Cornell group to which Neisser belongs are intellectual descendants of the pre-war Gestalt psychologists, who held that a perceived object is not merely the sum of all its parts. Neisser points to the richness of the visual clues from the environment, to an essentially constructive role of the brain in seeing and to the need for a 'pre-attentive process'. Sutherland, in his approach to perception, emphasises the translation of the information from the eye into abstract, descriptive rules. Broadbent, as we saw, stresses the brain's need to shed information and to attend to what seems to concern it.

As in other aspects of brain function, the processes of vision are sufficiently rich and complex for many disparate opinions to find their place. And the outsider can note them as converging on the single idea that we never see the world just as it is registered in the eye – as patches of colour and scribbles of lines. We select features from what we see and make a rapid succession of 'models' of the world in our minds. Paradoxically, we therefore see the world more clearly and usually more reliably than we should do if the eye were simply a camera.

Tricking the brain

'Optical illusions' is a misleading term for those little diagrams that surprise us by deceiving us, if it implies that the eye is foolish. In most cases the mind, not the eye, is outwitted. For Richard Gregory, lately of Edinburgh University, visual illusions (a safer term) provide proof of the brain's activity in making and selecting 'models' of the outside world from the information supplied by the eye. One of his experiments suggested this was the case for a very well-known illusion:

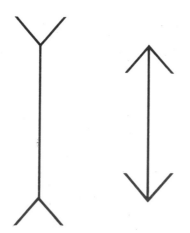

Why does the left-hand line appear longer than the right-hand one, when a simple check will show them to be the same length?

Of the possible reasons, Gregory preferred this one: we picture the left-hand figure as a perspective drawing of the far corner of a room or box, while the right-hand figure looks like a near corner. When the brain has arrived at this decision, it makes allowance for the fact that distant things usually look small, and concludes that the left-hand upright must be really quite big. Gregory obtained evidence for this explanation, using ingenious equipment in which people saw the figures in a mirror, as if suspended in space, and could measure how far away they thought the figures were. He also showed how the error in judgement of distance depended on the angles of the 'fins'.

But what happens if you try the ordinary test on a Bushman who lives in a semicircular shelter and has little experience of boxes? In the late 1950s, American anthropologists made a comparison between African tribesmen and American suburbanites, with some other nationalities thrown in for good measure. They found that the Americans were more readily tricked by the illusion than were the others unaccustomed to a world made with carpenters' squares. Our clues about perspective evidently depend on our experience.

The rural Africans were usually more prone to another kind of visual illusion:

The 'perspective' explanation for why many people believe the vertical line to be longer is that they imagine it as a path receding from them towards the horizon. Marshall Segal and his colleagues, who carried out these international comparisons, predicted that people living an outdoor life in a spacious environment would fall for the illusion more readily than would the American city-dwellers. They went on to say that others, living in a rain forest or a canyon, might be less susceptible to the

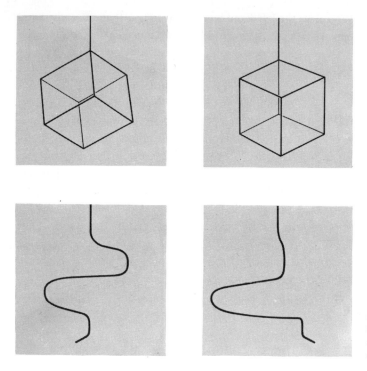

A cube remains obviously a cube as it rotates but an irregularly bent wire seems to change shape as it turns.

illusion. And so it turned out. Farmers in the plains of Uganda succumbed more readily to the illusion than did the Americans, while tribesmen who lived in forest clearings or among mountains were relatively immune.

Sometimes the brain fails to find a 'model' for what it sees. In another demonstration, Gregory projected the shadows of rotating shapes on to a flat screen and asked helpers what they made of them. When the shape was the framework of a cube, the viewer simply saw a cube rotating. It was hard to be certain which way round it was turning, so that it seemed to go now one way, now the other. But there was never any difficulty in seeing it always as a cube, and this perception remained even when several sides of the cube were cut out.

When the rotating shape was meaningless, just an irregularly bent piece of wire, the impression changed dramatically. The viewer could neither form a constant picture of the object nor even see it as something rotating. Instead, the shadow seemed like a dancing snake, continuously changing in shape. We have evidently no 'models' in our heads for meaningless bends – why should we?

Studies in the tricks of human vision became important in the US programme of manned spaceflight, which called for rendezvous and docking operations. A person driving on the ground towards an objective has plenty of clues about distance

from the general scene as well as from the target itself; in space,

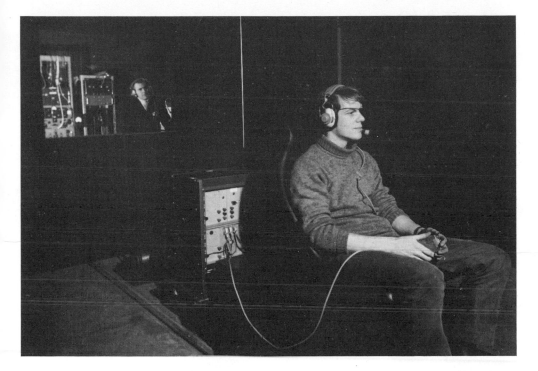

In this chair mounted on rails, at the University of Edinburgh, a man has to control the diameter of a circle projected on a screen in front of him, as he moves back and forth. Darkness and the lack of other clues adversely affect his performance as shown by the experiments of Richard Gregory and his colleagues.

these clues are lacking. Gregory and his colleagues undertook a series of experiments, including one in which a man sat in a moving chair in a dark tunnel looking at shapes at the far end. It soon became clear that the visual judgement of the astronauts would be highly unreliable in a rendezvous, a finding that was borne out in flight. Electronic aids became essential for manoeuvring.

A colleague of Gregory's in Edinburgh, Christopher Longuet-Higgins, recently made a robot called Fido, with an internal 'model' of the world. It consists of a trolley which can be moved by hand on a table-top. This remarkable device has so keen a sense of where it is that, whenever it is driven near the edge of the table, it sounds an alarm bell, just in time. The suspicious visitor looks in vain for eyes in the robot, or for sensors around the robot or around the table edge, and he deduces that some very clever electronics is at work inside the machine. Then Longuet-Higgins turns Fido over and reveals a joke which is rather more than a joke.

The computer consists primarily of a battery, a bell and a rectangular piece of cardboard. The simplest possible arrangement of internal wheels shifts the cardboard around in step with the movements of the trolley. When the trolley approaches the edge of the table, the position of the cardboard allows a contact to close, which rings the bell. The piece of cardboard, the same shape as the table but scaled down, is Fido's 'model' of the 173 world, a perfectly fair analogy to a blind man's internal 'model' of his bedroom, or even to our visual 'models' of familiar shapes.

Some further drawings show, far better than any words of mine, with just what force and conviction the brain selects a visual model and, having made its choice, reinforces it. There is the well-known vase which becomes a pair of faces.

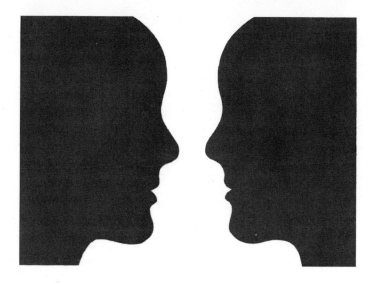

The first point to notice is that you flip decisively from one model to another. It is hard to compromise or to see the picture complete as two faces kissing the vase – a most unlikely contingency that would demand more visual evidence than is available here. Secondly, the flipping is partly but not wholly under conscious control. The relative strength of the models is a factor; once you have spotted the figures in Masson's landscape, below, it may become very difficult to see the landscape clearly at all.

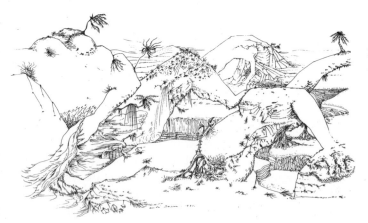

La Martinique, *a drawing by André Masson.*

A third point about the vase is that, when you flip over to it, the white may seem to become physically brighter, creating imaginary edges at the top and bottom where the vase contrasts with the apparently duller white of the rest of the page. The brain is reinforcing its conviction. The effect is clearer still when you interpret the strange pattern shown above; you may also experience an inward 'thump' of satisfaction when you see what it is.

Short step to the mind's eye

Gone is the old, crude idea that the connection from the sense organ to the brain is like a string, a tug on which rings a particular bell in the head. Not only does analytical processing, of the kind done by Hubel and Wiesel's feature detectors, transform the information; we now also see that the perceptive mind actively influences what it perceives. Compared with sight, our other senses are less thoroughly explored but they, too, supply evidence of mental intervention in processes formerly regarded as automatic.

An effect of hearing very like the flip-over from vase to faces (in the figure opposite) was found by Richard Warren and Richard Gregory in 1958. When a single tape-recorded word is repeated over and over again: 'rest, rest, rest, rest, rest . . .' a moment may come when the listener suddenly starts hearing a different word, not casually but emphatically. It might, in this example, be 'stress' or 'Esther'. The experiment suggests that the pattern-recognition processes at work in hearing are very like those in seeing.

In 1970 Warren, who is from the University of Wisconsin, Milwaukee, reported another effect. As a matter of everyday experience, occasional coughs or noises are not at all troublesome when we are listening to someone talking. Other experimenters showed that people could not report accurately when, during a sentence, an intrusive noise occurred. Warren finds that they cannot do so even if part of a word is completely eliminated. He took a recording of the sentence: 'The state governors met with their respective legi(s)latures convening in the capital city.' He cut out the portion at and around the 175 bracketed 's' and replaced it by a loud recorded cough of the same duration ($\frac{1}{8}$ second).

Warren played the tape to twenty students and gave them a typewritten copy of the sentence to mark with the position of the cough. Only ten of them thought the cough came during the word 'legislature' and 19 students denied that any sound was missing from the sentence. Warren repeated the experiment, using a tone instead of a cough, and the results were much the same. In hearing we perceive whole words and can restore missing sounds, just as in seeing we can imagine details that are missing from a sketch.

The brain's manufacture, from the information coming into the eye, of the 'models' of the outside world that we actually see is a formidable enterprise. It is inwardly recognisable as a very important mental operation which guides our actions. But the same mechanism also provides a basis for thought, using mental images, whether recalled or invented. It turns out that imagination, in its literal sense of making images in our heads, makes full use of the brain's organisation for the simplest tasks of looking and seeing.

Lee Brooks's experiments in Canada show conflict when the same brain mechanisms have to be used for memory and imagination at the same time as for action. In (1) a person has to remember what a block letter F looks like and go around it, responding 'yes' when a corner is at the extreme top or bottom, and 'no' when it is at an intermediate level. It is more difficult to give the answers by pointing than by speaking them. In (2), where a memorised sentence has to be similarly checked for the occurrence of nouns, speaking is more difficult than pointing.

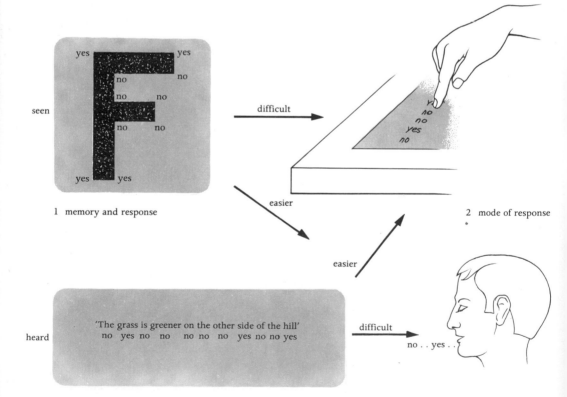

1 memory and response

2 mode of response

Purely mental images, vivid or sketchy according to the individual, can be conjured up in remembering, or when we have dreams or hallucinations. Ulric Neisser marshals the evidence that mental images come from just the same brain mechanisms as do the images of 'real' seeing. One is the fact that eye movements recorded during dreaming sometimes relate precisely to what the dreamer reports that he was looking at in his dream. Another is the subjective impression, when you are asked to think how many windows your house has, that you scan mental images of the house essentially as you would if you were inspecting it in reality.

Particularly striking evidence of a common brain mechanism comes from an experiment by Lee Brooks of McMaster University in Ontario. Brooks put volunteers in a situation in which they had to try both to use their visual imaginations and to see at the same time. They had to point, in a simple list, to a word describing one feature of a shape which they had seen previously. It turned out to be quite difficult, considerably more so than simply uttering the word, apparently because remembering the shape and looking at the list were competing for the same brain mechanism.

Even in the fully conscious state, mental images can be markedly different from anything ever seen in reality. For example, I can invite you to imagine a cobra in your bath. Plainly you will draw on your brain's stock of visual 'models' for your bath and for cobras, in making this little mental composition. But plainly, too, it is no supernatural leap from here to the ability of artist or engineer or schizophrenic to imagine forms not seen since the world began.

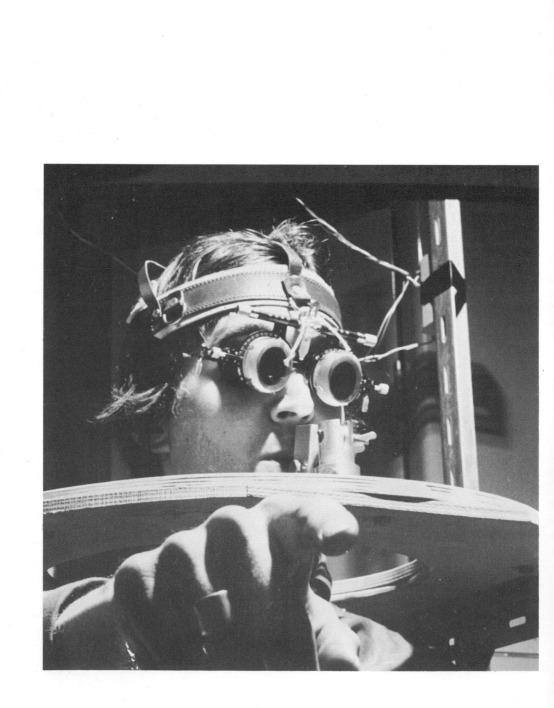

Hand and Eye

Abundant connections between different parts of the brain are needed for co-operation of hand and eye in learning and in creative work. But the simplest deliberate action raises questions of will, foresight and motive, for which the front of the brain may supply some of the answers.

Goggles for research in the psychology of vision. In this case, at the University of Sussex, the goggles contain half-prisms which produce a break between top and bottom of the scene.

How prisms displace the visual world.

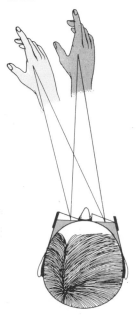

In the mid-nineteenth century the founder of the modern study of vision, Hermann von Helmholtz, started a fashion for peculiar spectacles that continues till now. He showed that a man seeing the world through a wedge-shaped prism would at first reach wrongly for an object but gradually come to aim more correctly. When the prism was removed, the man's vision was so adapted that he misreached in the opposite direction. By wearing prisms in front of his eyes, a man can distort his vision, shifting the scene to left or right, or up or down. Mirrors will reverse and re-angle the view; little telescopes can turn the world upside-down. In 1897 an American, George Stratton, lived for a week with an inverting telescope in front of one eye, with the other masked. By the end of that time he said he was seeing almost normally.

Although such experiments have long been popular with psychologists, they have won added significance in the past few years, especially through research by Richard Held and his colleagues, first at Brandeis University and recently at the Massachusetts Institute of Technology. Held has found that adaptation to the distorted view of the world, produced by wearing prisms, occurs only if the 'victim' has the opportunity to make active movements and observe their effects.

Held's volunteer, in a typical experiment, sits with one arm strapped to a board which is pivoted below the elbow, so that the hand can swing to left or right. He looks at his hand, which is visually shifted to one side by a prism. If he now moves his hand to and fro, he adapts within half an hour. Pointing tests show that he can fully compensate for the effect of the prism. But if, instead of moving his arm himself, he leaves it limp and lets the experimenter swing it for him, no adaptation occurs.

179

Similarly, a man wearing prism goggles adapts if he is free to walk about, while another man who is pushed in a wheelchair over the same route does not. Seeing and moving evidently depend on a joint map-making mechanism in the brain. You cannot launch your hand correctly to touch a coffee cup unless you see where the cup is standing. Conversely, you cannot learn to see correctly, as a child, or a goggle-wearer, unless you are free to touch cups, or otherwise explore with the limbs. The existence of such an interconnected system explains some strange effects in people who acquire sight after a lifetime of blindness.

Richard Gregory tells of such a man in Britain. This patient, 'SB', saw for the first time at the age of 52, after corneal grafting. He had led an active life and had explored the world by touch. He quickly learned to use his eyes, but a bias persisted towards objects he had explored by touch. A striking sign of this was the way he drew pictures of buses. He knew buses well by touch, inside and outside, naturally excepting the driver's cab and the motor compartment. Six months after the operation, SB could draw a neat picture of a double-decker bus – but the front of the bus was still missing.

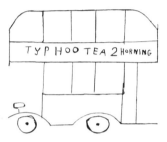

A man blind from birth, who acquired his sight, drew this picture of a bus six months after his operation. He left out the lower front, apparently because he had never explored it by touch while he was blind.

The idea that the sense of touch educates vision is a very old one, going back at least to Bishop Berkeley in the eighteenth century. It would be wrong not to point out that this apparent dependence of sight on touch is challenged in other modern research. For example, Charles and Judith Harris in experiments at the University of Pennsylvania also performed tests with distorting prisms, but they deduced that their volunteers came to believe that their hands were where they appeared to be: seeing was dominating touch. Again, a famous demonstration by Eleanor Gibson of Cornell University showed that babies shrank back from a 'visual cliff', a glass-covered pit which they could see but had never explored in any way.

In 1969, Martin Steinbach of Held's group extended the known powers of co-operation of hand and eye to include smooth tracking of the hand by the eye, on the basis of internal signals. He recorded the eye movements of people trying to follow a rapidly swinging spot of light, which flashed intermittently. They were not very successful. Indeed, they did not even have the impression of a moving target; lights seemed to flash on and off at different positions, with no apparent motion. But Steinbach also had them following the flashing spot when its position always corresponded to the position of the middle finger, with the arm on a pivoted board. Whether a man moved his own arm rapidly to and fro, or the experimenter swung it for him, the eye tracked the moving spot almost perfectly.

Second seeing

One of the most curious of the experiments with prisms was done a few years ago by Ivo Kohler of Innsbruck. It turns out to have foreshadowed an important new finding about brain mechanisms. If a prism covers only the top half of the field of view, a vertical line such as a flagpole appears broken, the upper part being shifted to right or left. When he has grown used to the prism, a man can point accurately towards objects in either the upper (shifted) or the lower (unshifted) scene. As a result, he locates both parts of the flagpole in exactly the same direction. The brain system dealing with the judgement of

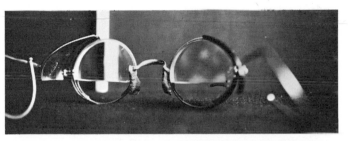

Kohler's half-prism spectacles greatly distort the vision, as in the scene below. But a man who becomes accustomed to them can point correctly to different parts of a vertical object even though he still sees it broken.

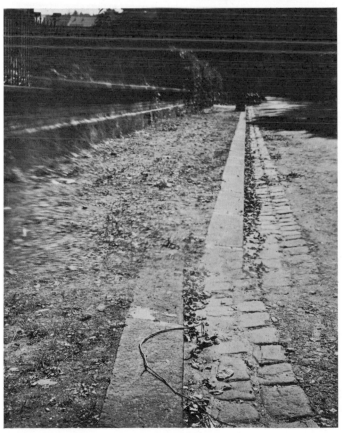

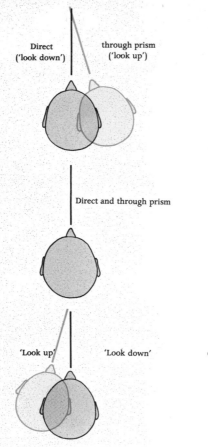

Direct
('look down')

through prism
('look up')

First day

Direct and through prism

Last day

'Look up'

'Look down'

Glasses removed

Effects of prisms in the upper field of view only. At first they cause an apparent displacement when the wearer looks up. After a time, the brain corrects for that effect, but when the prisms are removed there is an apparent displacement the other way in the upper field of view.

direction and guidance of the hand has fully compensated for the distortion produced by the prism. Yet the system dealing with shape has not compensated – the flagpole still looks broken!

The seeing mechanisms at the back of the brain detect the features and shapes of visible objects, as described in Chapter 9 in connection with the celebrated experiments of Hubel and Wiesel. But in that process, the brain seems to shed information about exactly in what direction the object lies. For the judgement of distance, comparisons of the same shape seen with the two eyes are made in the back of the brain. But one of the qualities of the 'complex' cells discovered by Hubel and Wiesel in the visual cortex is that they register a shape-feature regardless of its exact position in the field of view. But could such a system be efficiently organised to know exactly where the object is? Doubts on this score led Richard Held to argue that there must be a completely different visual system concerned with position rather than shape. This system would be especially important as an aid to movement, such as the launching of the hand towards an objective.

182

Deliberate damage to animal brains provides evidence for a second seeing mechanism, very much involved in the control of orientation and movement. Monkeys who have forfeited the first seeing region at the back of the brain lose their natural ability to recognise objects and patterns, but they are still able to turn their eyes and head towards an isolated visible object and to reach in the right direction for it.

Gerald Schneider at MIT announced, in 1970, the most convincing demonstation of the existence of two distinct visual systems. Golden hamsters have, in Schneider's phrase, an 'insatiable propensity to search for sunflower seeds', and these were the animals he chose for experiments in which two different kinds of damage were done to the brain. Conclusions from informal tests, in which the animals looked for sunflower seeds held in the hand, were confirmed and elaborated in mechanised test situations. Some of the animals lost the use of the visual cortex at the back of the brain, the region investigated by Hubel and Wiesel. Like the monkeys just mentioned, these hamsters failed tests of pattern recognition, but they would still raise or turn their heads towards a moving object.

In another group of hamsters, the visual cortex was left undamaged, but a quite different part of the brain was disconnected – the 'little hill', the superior colliculus, on either side of

A region on each side of the brain stem known as the superior colliculus seems to provide a separate visual system for judging direction, rather than shape.

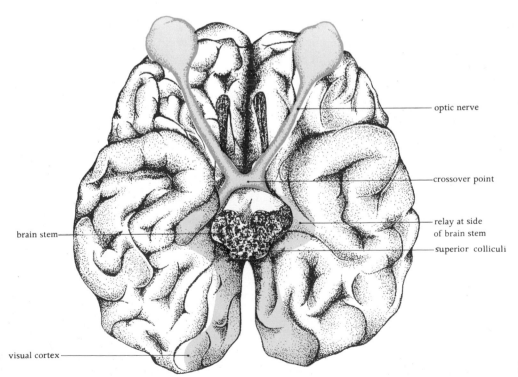

optic nerve

crossover point

relay at side
of brain stem

superior colliculi

brain stem

visual cortex

183

the brain stem. These animals acted almost as if they were blind, and showed no response in the tests of directed head-turning. Yet they were perfectly capable of distinguishing between doors marked with vertical and horizontal stripes, and learning to go through the correct door to obtain water. Unless there is something very unusual about the hamster, human beings, too, presumably possess separate visual systems concerned with direction-finding and located in the middle of the brain.

Will intrudes

The exercise of will, one of the most important components of the human mind, seems at first thought to be too personal, abstract or esoteric a process to pin down as a brain mechanism. Certainly, no one can yet say by what machinery he makes a decision to act and is conscious of making it. Does the will therefore remain a high-level mental activity concerning which the philosopher suffers no competition from the brain researchers? Second thoughts may persuade you that manifestations of will in action may not be too difficult to identify, in the routines of the brain. 'Did you jump or did you fall?' The subjective fact that the sensations are very different in the two cases gives a clue to how some brain scientists set about distinguishing the voluntary from the involuntary act.

Our high-level mental activities are likely to be traced to the systems deep in the brain which routinely integrate perception and movement. An obvious example is the co-operation of hand and eye – the combination of skills that reached such a peak with the emergence of man as to be a key element of human nature and human achievement. It is the origin of our immense technical ability, from the manufacture of stone arrowheads to making music and steering spacecraft.

The control of the muscles is no lowly, mechanical task. No one would be advised to try telling a craftsman or an airline pilot that his hands act mindlessly, nor would a surgeon or a pianist readily concede that his fingers are self-governing machines. Effective movement, as contrasted with the limb-flailing of a baby, a dreamer or an epileptic, requires the exercise of will. Even when a skill has become a routine, looked after by the little brain, the cerebellum, the appropriate programme is switched on 'at will' – on instructions from a higher centre. Attempts to explain the simplest deliberate movement (waving to a friend, say) make little headway without allowing for will.

Experimenters are understandably cautious about invoking ideas like will and purpose. Some responses, like snatching back the finger from a hot surface, do not even involve the brain. The possibility, advanced in all seriousness by able men, that a human being is nothing but a complicated bundle of simple reflexes, needs to be tested. In an experiment more than 30 years ago, Delos Wickens had human volunteers sit with the palm down and one finger slightly crooked, touching an electric contact. A wire on the wrist completed the electric circuit and Wickens switched on a mild current half a second after a warning sound.

The volunteer quickly learned to straighten the finger at the sound, so lifting it and escaping the shock. When this habit was well established, the hand was turned palm up, with the back of the same finger touching the contact. Most volunteers responded to the warning sound by bending the finger, reversing what they had done before. The layman may think this was a ludicrous experiment, merely proving that human beings are not generally as stupid as the experimenter; but, of course, Wickens was trying to help establish why we are not stupid. What his volunteers learned was not a crude muscle response but a strategy, with the goal of avoiding the shock.

Without a goal, or more typically a rapid succession of goals, the brain can co-ordinate a movement no better than a ship's helmsman can steer without a course being set. All other complex animals, besides humans, must possess will at least in its essentials of decision-making and anticipating consequences. There is no way of telling whether a dog is conscious of any exercise of will, but he must be capable of some kind of commanding or programming mechanism if he is to chase cats in a well-organised manner.

Will must figure prominently in the details of the control of movement. A hurdler does not merely decide to leap – he decides rather precisely what paths his body and limbs should follow. These decisions allow the brain to compute detailed programmes for all the relevant muscles. The action is then governed by the mechanisms which compare the actual state of the muscles at any instant with the programmed state, and make the necessary corrections. In practice, the eyes are usually very much involved.

Back to the front

Earlier, in Chapter 6, the front of the brain was called an unknown universe, but the search for will leads us back to it. Mild electric stimulation of the frontal lobes, when a human being's skull is open for surgery, usually produces no activity in the patient to compare with the rather dramatic results from   185 stimulation of other parts of the brain. But one striking effect is as follows. If the side of one frontal lobe is stimulated, the patient will automatically turn his head away, but his eyes continue looking straight ahead. In other words the eyes turn in their sockets to just the extent needed to compensate for the head movement. Hans-Lukas Teuber, of MIT, takes this rather complex response as evidence that the front of the brain assists in mechanisms of compensation.

You can easily prove to yourself that unconscious compensation is at work all the time in the brain. First, glance from side to side and satisfy yourself that normal eye movements do not move the world – by which I mean that you have no impression that the room you are sitting in is moving, rather than your eyes. This is so natural a state of affairs that you may not understand what I am driving at. But now close one eye and press (very gently please) on the side of the other eye with a finger; just enough to make the eye wobble a little.

Then you will see what I mean: the world appears to move. The implication of this simple experiment is quite profound. Whenever nerve signals go to our eyes to make them turn 'of their own accord', another signal must go simultaneously to the regions of the brain concerned with seeing. This signal says, in effect, 'Make allowance for a coming swing to the left, and hold the world still'. When you moved your eye with your finger you by-passed this early-warning system and took your seeing by surprise.

Teuber has a name for the alerting signal that goes from the movement areas of the brain to the sense areas: a 'corollary discharge'. What makes Teuber's views most interesting, in our search for the familiar mind in the unfamiliar universe of brain cells, is that he sees in the corollary discharge, or warning signal, a scientific approach to the notion of will.

Teuber says that a 'voluntary' or 'self-produced' (or 'willed') movement is distinguished from an 'automatic' or 'reflex' movement because it involves a corollary discharge. When the front of the brain is out of action the powers of voluntary control are impaired: the patient may still be able to foresee a course of events, yet not be able to picture himself in relation to those events.

Consider another aspect of our little experiment. When you poked your finger towards your eye, to move it, warning signals were flying around. To the brain area concerned with finger and cheek touch: 'Expect contact'. To the movement area in charge of the operation: 'As soon as that contact is reported, stop moving at once; then advance very slowly and steadily to put pressure on the eyeball. In event of pain, with-

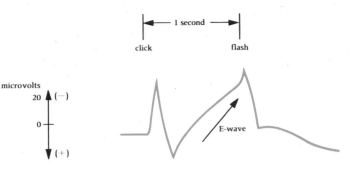

The expectancy wave, a build-up of a negative electric voltage across the front of the brain when a person is expecting something to happen imminently; it discharges when the awaited event occurs. (After Grey Walter)

draw instantly.' It is unlikely that you were conscious of working all that out, though quite probable that you were aware of the need for caution. Thus does the simple idea of the corollary discharge quickly grow into a mechanism for planning and controlling complex actions and for foreseeing their consequences.

Teuber's theory of the corollary discharge is not proved. The presumed pathways for carrying the warning signals from the frontal lobes to the sense areas are certainly not conspicuous in the brain. And, obviously, the will is more than just a broadcasting system. To supply a running commentary on the expected consequences of willed movements is not the same thing as initiating them. Nevertheless, Teuber's idea is enticing and he finds support for it in some of the consequences of bullet wounds in the frontal lobes, including difficulties in judging orientation in a tilted chair and in relating information acquired by touch to visual information.

Using very different methods to examine the effects of injury to the front of the brain, Alexander Luria in Moscow has come to conclusions so similar that Teuber calls the agreement 'simply astonishing'. Luria believes that the frontal lobes enable the organism to behave in a manner that conforms with the effect produced by its actions. In his view, this part of the brain is very much involved both with the motor strip and with the deeper-lying regions of the brain concerned with the state of the body. But Luria still emphasises that the frontal lobes are the most difficult region of the brain to investigate.

The silliness syndrome

Like others who know these cases, Luria relates many strange performances by patients with extensive damage to the front of the brain: the man who went on striking a match when it was already alight; the man in the carpenter's shop who planed a piece of wood completely through and continued planing the bench; the man who asked to leave the hospital and was shown the door of the room, but walked into a cupboard instead. Among Soviet war-wounded, fewer than one in ten of those with frontal-lobe damage were able to master a task in occupational therapy, compared with four in ten with injuries in other parts of the brain.

The characteristic difficulty is in working systematically through a succession of actions to achieve a goal. There may also be much less determination to conquer a disability than in patients with other brain injuries. And when a frontal-lobe patient examines a realistic picture he is likely to give a very bizarre opinion of what it depicts. A death-bed scene may be described as a wedding, because of a white dress, or as someone suffering from a cold, because of a handkerchief. Such responses to pictures seemed so highly characteristic of severe injury to the front of the brain that Luria and his colleagues decided to investigate them more fully.

They recorded the eye movements while patients were looking at a picture and were asked questions about it. Examples of what the tests revealed are shown opposite. When a normal person studies a picture he looks for significant details; when asked a question, he will search for appropriate information. For example, the question 'How old are the people in the picture?' will prompt an examination of faces; asked whether the family is rich or poor, the normal person examines the furnishing of the room. The eye movements of a frontal-lobe patient looking at the same picture may, by contrast, be completely chaotic and aimless, influenced neither by the structure of the picture nor by the questions asked.

Eye movements recorded in tests done in Moscow, as a normal person (left-hand tracks) and a patient with severe damage to the right frontal lobe (right-hand tracks) explore the same picture, without instruction and in response to questions. The patient shows little organisation of eye movements. (Data from Luria)

The front of the brain does not yield up its secrets easily but other clues to its activities come from recordings of electric brain waves in that region of the head. From the Burden Institute in Bristol, W. Grey Walter and his colleagues reported in 1964 the discovery of the 'expectancy wave', or E-wave. In their experiment, a person knew, when he heard a click, that one second later a light would flash and then he had to press a button.

Electrodes on the person's scalp picked up the E-wave in such circumstances, from the front of the head. First the click produced a brief jerk in the record; then, during the ensuing second, a negative electric voltage grew on the front of the brain, reaching a peak at the moment of the flash and then suddenly discharging as the expectation was fulfilled. In Walter's opinion, the E-wave is a sign of the brain preparing for 'synchronous and economical action'.

In the Institute of Higher Nervous Activity in Moscow, also in the mid-1960s, M. I. Livanov reported other discoveries

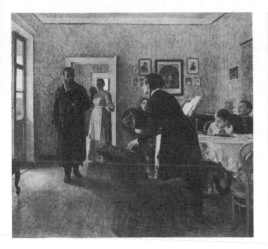

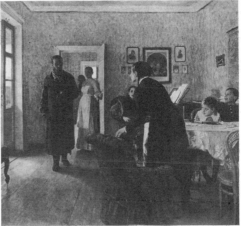

No question

No question

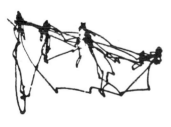

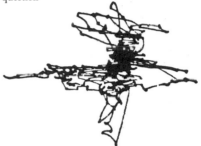

How old
are the people in the picture?

How old
are the people in the picture?

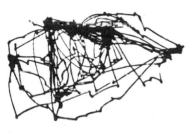

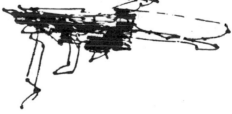

Try to memorise the clothing
the people are wearing

Try to memorise the clothing
the people are wearing

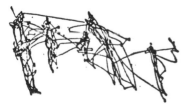

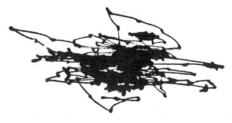

concerning synchronous electrical activity in the frontal lobes. He used a large number of electrodes simultaneously to record the electric waves at many different points over the scalp. When a normal person was sitting quietly, the records from different parts of the brain were just a jumble of disconnected waves. But when he was asked to multiply two two-figure numbers (44 times 68, say) the electric activity became synchronous in parts of the brain, especially across the frontal lobes, as if these were among the areas of the brain working on the problem.

This evidence of the engagement of the frontal lobes in normal mental activity was interesting enough, but Livanov proceeded to make the same sort of records in abnormal circumstances. He found that a tranquilliser drug, chlorpromazine, markedly reduced the common rhythms in the frontal lobes. By contrast, a mental patient suffering from a delirious form of schizophrenia showed feverish synchronous activity even when resting. A patient with damage to the frontal lobes showed no such patterns even when given a mental task.

We need not suppose that the frontal lobes are where we actually make decisions. That may occur, if indeed it can be said to happen anywhere in particular, deep in the mid-brain. The front of the brain is perhaps more like a trusted adviser who handles public relations and planning. One way of looking at the clinical evidence is to see the frontal lobes supplying 'nous', intelligence of a non-intellectual kind; moria, or 'silliness', is the frequent consequence of damage in those regions. In the opinion of some experts, the frontal lobes are also a principal source of the conscious feeling, 'Here I am'. That is plausible enough, in view of the evident role of the front of the brain in helping us to picture ourselves in relation to ongoing events.

Scrappy knowledge

The last few chapters have sampled current lines of research to tell how functions are allocated through the human brain and how, in detail, some of those functions are carried out. We have looked at the workings of individual brain cells not just as technicalities but as living participants in vastly elaborate analytical machinery, for example in the cerebellum and the visual cortex. For other of the higher functions, such as visual perception and imagination, we have had to rely on psychological evidence of procedures adopted by the brain, instead of attempting to trace the circuits involved. That is what we shall have to do increasingly, in the rest of the book, as we change course to deal particularly with some of the grander issues involving the brain as a whole.

Even so, everything that has gone before could be said to be thoroughly misleading, if it gives the impression that the brain has surrendered its secrets and the scientists are just mopping up the details. Research workers are opportunists and so are reporters: we like to tell a good story and to pass over topics about which there is nothing to say. I have tried to make plain where speculation has to stand in for great volumes of knowledge which we do not possess – in writing about the will, for example. But perhaps I should emphasise that those gaps in our knowledge span most of the functions of the brain, and especially the systems of connection, co-ordination and interpretation which are the essence of the active brain. Our knowledge is scrappy, to say the least.

But there is no reason for pessimism. Fragmented though it is, the knowledge is growing quite rapidly. What is more, it is fitting together in most encouraging ways. In the cerebellum, for example, acquaintance with its general function, mapping of detailed connections, functional studies with micro-electrodes, knowledge about how brain cells work, and mathematical theory, have all combined – yielding a very persuasive story about how the cerebellum remembers to carry out an action. Furthermore that advance, combined with the discovery of the part of the brain responsible for the implanting of long-term memory, makes the whole question of memory storage in the brain seem much less intractable than it did even a few years ago.

As we turn now to the great issues about man's special powers, about individuality and environment and about the origin of consciousness, we shall not completely desert the surgeons, the animal experimenters, or the men with electrodes and test tubes. They have vital and provocative information to give. Wherever possible, we shall want to pinpoint systems and events in the brain associated with these big questions. But other men of learning have their points of view – linguists, educational psychologists, nutritionists and philosophers. The issues have implications far beyond the simple urge of the scientist to find out new things. What follows bears upon human self-esteem, on policies for bringing up children, on politics in general and on the future of man as chief tenant of the planet earth.

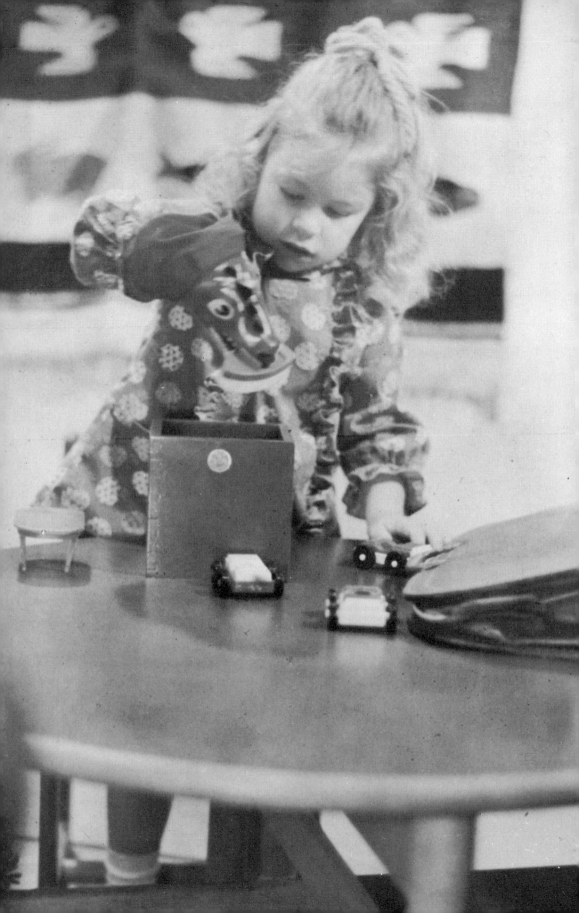

Part Three: Mind Emergent

11   The Human Powers

Despite some promising attempts to communicate with chimpanzees, language remains the most obvious faculty distinguishing us from other animals. How we achieve it is one of the liveliest of current questions. Some other currents of human achievement seem to flow from ordinary brain mechanisms.

Michelle and the dragon. Reasearch into the way children acquire language requires little equipment, but much patience.

In the William James Hall at Harvard a young graduate student and a three-year-old girl take turns in using a toy dragon to rearrange a box of toys. 'Dragon, put the boat in,' says Michelle and on her little 'the' hangs an argument. The student is examining a fine point about Michelle's powers of language, in one of the latest in a series of studies led by Roger Brown, into how children learn to talk. Student and child play supporting roles in one of the major intellectual dramas of our time. The principals are near at hand.

In that same tower block at Harvard, named in honour of the most celebrated American psychologist of the 1890s, the best known of contemporary experimental psychologists enjoys an active retirement amid the pigeon empire that he founded. Burrhus F. Skinner wears the mantle of Ivan Pavlov. The proposition that all conduct is a matter of conditioned reflexes Skinner saved from early disrepute by enlarging the scope of conditioning. A typical Skinnerian explanation of human powers is the following: 'As we write a paragraph, we create an elaborate chain of verbal stimuli which alter the probabilities of other words to follow.' And for him, language is a faculty acquired, like anything else, by trial and error in a context of stimulus, response and reward for success.

Just along the Charles River from Harvard, in a cramped office in one of the tattier buildings of the Massachusetts Institute of Technology, you will find Noam Chomsky, Skinner's fiercest opponent. To the American public he is conspicuous as a leader of the anti-war movement, but to the world's academics he is the man who found hidden depths in the most casual human utterances and worked out a new theory of grammar. Of most previous approaches to the human mind

Chomsky says: 'We tend too easily to assume that explanations must be transparent and close to the surface.'

Along with a couple of apes living beyond the Rockies, these are some of the participants in the drama. As it involves equipment like toy dragons, research in linguistics lacks the polished splendour of space rocketry. There is little here to compare with the accelerators and telescopes whereby physicists and astronomers are uncovering the nature and history of the universe we inhabit. But in this other great search, for the mind of man, nothing is more important for grasping the realities of human nature than the inquiry into the origins of language. Our powers of language, more decisively than any of our other talents, distinguish us mentally from the other animals.

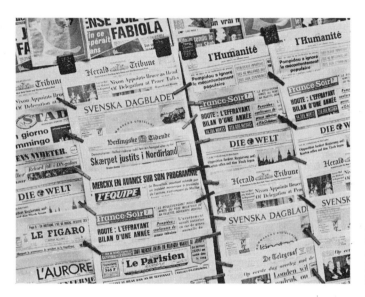

According to Chomsky and other linguists, behind the obvious differences in the thousands of human languages there lies a common structure.

Mapping the language areas

A language lump in the human brain was found in 1968, by Norman Geschwind and Walter Levitsky at Boston University, during careful examination of a hundred brains obtained at post-mortem. In right-handed individuals, and in nearly half the left-handed too, the powers of language are almost entirely contained within the left side of the brain. But tradition had it that there was no visible difference between the left brain and the right. A few researchers had questioned this view, though inconclusively.

Geschwind and Levitsky found that, when they exposed the top of the temporal lobes to full view, the difference between right and left was often conspicuous. In two-thirds of the cases, a particular portion of the left temporal lobe was enlarged; the same portion was bigger on the right side in only one brain in nine. The newly-discovered lump occurs in a part of the brain identified a hundred years ago (by a German, Wernicke) as being involved in the higher analysis of speech sounds.

Pointing to areas of the brain especially involved in the use of language is no more an explanation of how they work than is a plan of the UN building an explanation of international politics. But that is how we must begin. At least it can be said that no feeling of over-simplification need arise from mapping the language areas of the brain.

Once again the disorders due to brain damage and the effects of electrical stimulation during brain operations are the prime

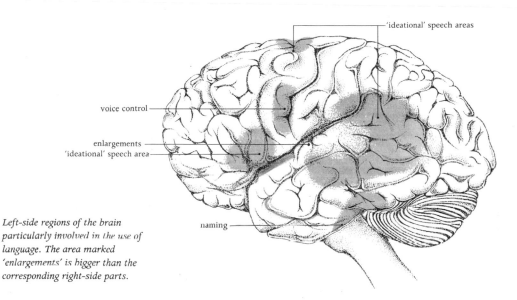

Left-side regions of the brain particularly involved in the use of language. The area marked 'enlargements' is bigger than the corresponding right-side parts.

sources of information. In practice, the loss of speech known as aphasia has a long history of investigation. Large parts of the left side of the brain were regarded as 'forbidden territory' for brain surgeons, for fear of causing aphasia, and this prohibition prompted Wilder Penfield and Lamar Roberts in Montreal to closer inquiry into which parts were really essential for speech. They were able, in the late 1950s, to offer some emphatic statements.

The most important area for speech is the hindmost, the so-called parieto-temporal area. Damage here can produce permanent loss of speech. In Penfield's view, this region of the roof of the brain interacts with his supposed 'higher' integrative region deep inside the brain, during the comprehension of speech and reading. Second in importance is a region lying further forward at the side of the brain, where damage produces long-lasting loss of speech. Eventually other parts of the brain may succeed in taking over its function, which seems to be that of preparing to make an utterance. Finally, there is an area at the top, the loss of which causes aphasia for only a few weeks.

These three areas on the left of the brain, Penfield and Roberts call 'ideational'. They are concerned with the content and meaning of language, in distinction from the part of the motor strip looking after the mechanics of voice control. Damage to the motor strip is less harmful, provided the corresponding area on the other side of the brain remains intact: there is a slurring of speech at first, which eventually clears up.

The practical use of language involves more areas than these. Alexander Luria, of Moscow, has made a special study of the many parts which come into play when a man writes what someone tells him – when, for example, you jot down an address given over the telephone. As with other manifestations of the human brain in action, this task seems so easy and familiar that its true complexity is not readily grasped.

A word enters the ear and its recognition is itself a formidable enough enterprise. The complex machinery of the snail-like cochlea of the inner ear converts a confused pattern of sound waves into a coded signal sent to the brain. The audible differences between words such as vine, wine, whine and Rhine are very slight, yet they are instantly distinguished, at least by an English speaker. The brain mechanisms for hearing and understanding words are, by the way, different from those for hearing and understanding music. One case in point was a patient of Luria's, the Russian composer Shebalin, who produced his best work after a stroke had robbed him of his ability to understand speech. The stroke was on the left side; music is usually dealt with on the right.

The critical acoustic area for the recognition process for words lies in the left temporal lobe; people injured there may be unable to distinguish 'b' from 'p', or 'd' from 't', and may be prevented from writing because they cannot think of the components of the words. The way people rely on saying the words to themselves was shown by spelling tests in a Russian school: when the children were told to keep their mouths wide open they made six times as many mistakes. Strikingly enough, Chinese children, whose words are pictorial rather than phonetic, are not affected in this way, and Chinese injured in the acoustic area do not lose their ability to write.

To set down words correctly, at least three other regions of the roof of the brain intervene before the signals go out from the motor strip to the fingers. One we have encountered before, in the case of the Russian soldier Z who lost his sense of direction. The normal ability to shape letters correctly depends on the internal map-making powers located high up and towards the back of the brain, in the parietal region. Patients injured here find reading and writing difficult and, when they do write, some of them unintentionally produce mirror-writing, running from right to left.

The task of putting letters and words together in the correct order involves the foremost of the 'ideational speech areas', low in the left of the brain and towards the front. Damage leaves patients unable to write (or speak) whole words, though able to produce individual letters or syllables. A still higher level of organisation is that supplied by the frontal lobes, the region generally associated with programming and planning. The handwriting of a frontal-lobe patient may show meaningless repetition of letters and words. Altogether, a large part of the left roof of the brain is involved in the 'simple act' of handwriting. Tests of handwriting can help to indicate just where damage exists on that side of the brain.

Grammar in the genes?

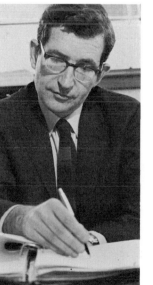

Noam Chomsky: 'We tend too easily to assume that explanations must be transparent.'

For some philosophers, the gift of language has been sufficient proof of the existence of the soul. In the seventeenth century, working in Holland, René Descartes pointed out that, although animals or automatic machines could utter speech-like sounds, they could not match even a human idiot in his capacity to arrange words into statements conveying his thoughts. Descartes' view was that this peculiarly human creative ability with language could not be explained by any machine-like system. In our own time, the first attempts at mechanising language, in using computers for the translation of foreign-language texts, have been an expensive failure. It seems impossible at present to make computers understand human language at any more profound level than the substitution of words from a dictionary.

Noam Chomsky works in the tradition of Descartes and he played a part in stopping the computer people and their patrons wasting more effort on this hopeless task. Unlike Descartes, or some readers of his own ideas, Chomsky is not suggesting a supernatural explanation for language – I have particularly pressed him on this point. But he does suspect that much more powerful science than we now possess will be needed, before we can fully relate language to physical processes in the brain, or explain the mind of man.

197

Chomsky's thesis packs together a number of points which should be separated for inspection, because some may be right while others may be wrong. His opposition to B. F. Skinner and the 'behaviourists', which he made plain in a celebrated review, is very noteworthy, but let us deal with outward conclusions rather than with academic in-fighting about philosophy and methods. At the other extreme from such polemics is Chomsky's own solid linguistic work, which presents a theoretical description that emphasises 'deep structure' and the enormously creative power of language as used by ordinary human beings.

He offers a universal grammar to which he thinks any human language must conform. As others have done before him, Chomsky looks below the surface structure of sentences. The sentence, 'A wise man is honest', breaks down, on the surface, into subject ('a wise man') and predicate ('is honest'). But it conceals an underlying proposition: 'a man is wise'. The importance of this apparently simple qualification emerges if you consider why 'A wisdom man is honest' is ungrammatical and 'A populous man is honest' is nonsense; the underlying propositions are wrong. An ambiguous sentence may be understood correctly only by appeal to underlying propositions: 'I know a taller man than Bill' – than Bill is, or than Bill knows?

In Chomsky's hands the deep structure becomes the agent for generating an infinite number of sentences, using transformational rules of great complexity to produce the surface structure of ordinary speech. From one underlying idea different, grammatically correct, sentences can emerge: 'The boy hit the ball', 'The boy hit the ball, didn't he?', or 'The ball was hit by the boy'. To account for the normal use of language Chomsky says we must attribute to both speaker and hearer, rules and mental operations of a very abstract nature.

Also in the Chomskyite package are other propositions which are really distinct. One is that his descriptive theory corresponds closely to how human beings actually use language. This is a crucial point which has been questioned. Donald Broadbent in Cambridge, England, compares Chomsky's linguistics with Euclid's geometry, as a great intellectual achievement, useful and beautiful, but not necessarily a description of natural phenomena. Euclid's geometry is misleading for navigators traversing the curved surface of the Earth. Chomsky's grammar certainly describes a body of utterances, but those utterances may nevertheless be produced by a quite different mechanism.

Following closely behind Chomsky's belief that his theory
tells how people actually use language is a second important

supposition that linguistic competence is inborn. The complex rules of language are mastered by young children, regardless of their intellectual rating, the literacy of their parents or the details of their experience. It is certainly hard to see how the children could manage it unless some of the principles are built into their brains by the genes of human heredity. The Skinnerian view sees the child born with only the most general mental powers, a 'clean slate' on which grammar is inscribed by experience. Against this rival proposition is the evidence that all normal children in all countries master their very different languages at just about the same ages and by essentially the same steps in grammar and vocabulary.

Thirdly, the human linguistic competence is unique, in Chomsky's view. By this he means more than the statement of the obvious, that humans talk and dogs don't. The uniqueness implies some qualitative difference between human beings and other animals – something more than having larger brains and subtler voices. And here we come back to Chomsky's war with the animal psychologists. How animals learn, reason and conduct themselves may tell us little or nothing about the way humans act, who think with the aid of words.

Some experimenters have tested the responses of ordinary people to ambiguous sentences of exactly the same kind discussed by Chomsky. For example: 'Our learning that John had won the race surprised him' – surprised whom, John or someone else? Housewives and sailors meeting this question, at the Applied Psychology Research Unit in Cambridge, gave it an average rating of 2.45, on the scale between 1 (definitely John) and 5 (definitely someone else).

As Chomsky says, that sentence is ambiguous. But he goes on to declare that a slightly different sentence, 'Learning that John had won the race surprised him', is not ambiguous – 'him' must refer to someone else, in accordance with transformational rules. The British people tested with these sentences were evidently less confident about the rules than Chomsky: their average rating was only 3.60, well short of the 5.00 required by the grammatical theory.

But the verdict on Chomsky's main points is more likely to come from the studies of young children, if anywhere. It is fairly obvious that a child is no passive listener and imitator. He will utter words that he has never heard an adult use – saying, for example, 'heared' instead of 'heard'. Such a mistake is a splendid demonstration of the intellect of a human infant. He is making his own theories about how language works and applying them with cheerful logic in new situations. He also has to master the irregularities and special usages of his native 199 language, at least to some extent, by trial and error. But even for that he has astonishing aptitude.

As Eric Lenneberg of Cornell University has found, there is a close relationship between development of controlled movement, maturing of brain tissue and emergence of language in a child. The tendency to speak is automatic. Lenneberg could not, for example, find any great difference in the rate or pattern of development of speech in normal babies of deaf parents, as compared with normal babies of normal parents.

Learning the rules

If Chomsky is right, he may transform our twentieth-century view of man and restore the Cartesian sense of inexplicable wonder in modern form. At least, he is a much-needed antidote to some acidulous psychological potions of recent vintage. But any dogma, including Chomsky's own, tends to oversimplify. It will be surprising if the evidence now being so earnestly sought does not, in the end, favour a view intermediate between Skinner's and Chomsky's. Whatever the outcome, human self-appraisal is at stake.

The toy dragon, mentioned at the outset, officiates in another example of the experiments now being done. 'Incredible delicacy' is Roger Brown's description of the use in English and other languages of the definite and indefinite articles, 'the' and 'a(n)'. His research student, Michael Maratsos, tests this usage in children aged 3 to $4\frac{1}{2}$ to see how competent they are,

Michael Maratsos' briefcase makes a hill in a story that tests a child's mastery of 'a' versus 'the'.

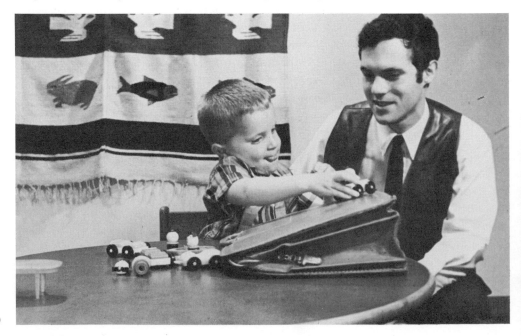

during this period when many of the oddities and illogicalities of language are being sorted out in their minds. He tells them stories, puts questions and persuades the children to ask for toys in a simple game.

The difference between 'Dragon wants a car' and 'Dragon wants the car' is superficially slight. But the correct usage depends on how many cars are available, on whether recent attention has been drawn to any special car and, generally, on what the speaker thinks the other person knows. There are supplementary rules: for example, the sun, the ground and the shops (local shops) are so well understood that they usually take 'the'; materials like 'soil' and 'toothpaste' rarely take 'a'. For the importance of the distinction in adult language, consider the effect of changing 'the' to 'a' in 'To be, or not to be: that is a question'.

Maratsos aims at informality, with everything a game or a story, in order that the children should think as little as possible about what they are saying. If pressed, children may perform worse than they really know how. Even so, errors do occur; it takes time for a child to develop the 'incredible delicacy'. Little Michelle (three years five months) says, correctly, 'Dragon, put the table in', where there is only one table available, but goes on to say, 'Dragon, put the dog in', although there are four dogs in sight. 'What dog?' Maratsos naturally asks. The object of his investigation is to find out about the basic competence of the child in handling 'the' and 'a', and how it matures around the age of four years, as the child's brain extracts the rules of language.

So how do people actually use language, and children acquire it? How much is in-built; how much is written by experience on the clean slate? The experiments mentioned illustrate the complexity of language and the fine points being tested, but they do not yet give any definite answer to these questions; nor do the many other investigations. George Miller of the Rockefeller University, a leading authority on the psychology of language, studies a variety of issues. One is the child's learning to use pronouns and passive sentences, which figure prominently in Chomsky's theory as 'transformations'; another is the way a person's store of words is organised, in thesaurus fashion, in the brain.

While keeping an open mind about how normal children acquire language, we can note a special area where Skinnerian methods of training certainly seem to produce favourable results. Autistic children are typically tragic youngsters, apparently of normal intelligence and vocal powers, who fail to communicate with other people; in particular, they fail to learn to talk. In the United States, Britain, Germany and else-where, psychiatrists have had successes in breaking the silence barrier by rewarding steps towards communication. In a fixed routine, the child is rewarded with sweets or ice-cream for meeting the gaze, for making a sound, for saying a word . . . and so on, through more elaborate use of language. Any pro-gress made in this direction seems to relieve whatever psychic reason for silence existed. Similar methods are also being tried with adult mental patients in whom silence is both a symptom of their disorder and a barrier to therapy.

One of Chomsky's contentions, noted earlier, is that language is a uniquely human faculty. Birds sing and monkeys squawk as a means of communication with their colleagues, and parrots can mimic human phrases, but these are nothing like creative language in the human sense. That animals may possess latent powers of language is a possibility to which we now turn.

Chatting with a chimpanzee

The real-life fable of Clever Hans gives a stern warning to any-one interpreting the conduct of animals in their dealings with humans. In Germany, more than 60 years ago, Clever Hans was a performing horse. He communicated by tapping his foot on the ground and by this means he exhibited amazing ability in reading, writing and arithmetic. Learned professors examined Clever Hans and declared that there was no deception; the horse could do all that was claimed for him. Then, one day, a sceptic named Oskar Pfungst insisted that Clever Hans be shown a question which no humans present could see. When that happened, the horse went on tapping his foot indefinitely. He waited in vain for the unconscious sign of expectancy that would tell him to stop because he had reached the right answer.

More genuine displays of problem-solving ability in animals figure in large numbers of experiments, where rats have to find their way through mazes, or other animals are faced with other tasks. The interpretation of these tests is a controversial busi-ness, particularly about the extent to which the animals have insight and reason resembling our own mental processes. It is only prudent to avoid imagining thought processes similar to what our own would be in the same situation, unless the evi-dence makes it inescapable, because we have no way of read-ing the animals' mental processes except through their visible conduct.

One of the classical experiments showing intellect in the chimpanzee was as follows. A chimpanzee chained to a tree could see a banana lying beyond his reach. Nearby was a stick which was, however, too short for reaching the banana and raking it in. Off to one side lay a longer stick, also out of the chimpanzee's immediate grasp, but near enough to be reached with the aid of the short stick. After some ineffective efforts to reach the banana with the short stick, the chimpanzee wandered about frustratedly until suddenly, with complete deliberation, he took the short stick, drew in the longer stick and then ran back with it to get the banana.

Rudimentary communication between man and animals is ancient. Even dogs, whose intellectual powers are small by human standards, learn to distinguish a few verbal commands. They can also make a few of their urges known to humans, for example bringing the leash as a cue for going for a walk. Men break into the natural communications within other species when they imitate mating calls or signs for decoy purposes.

Since 1945 a number of serious attempts have been made to establish richer dialogue between man and animal, in the tradition of St Francis and Dr Dolittle.

Chimpanzees were the obvious choice, being highly intelligent by non-human standards. When two American psychologists, K. J. and Caroline Hayes, attempted to teach a chimpanzee named Vicki to speak English, four words imperfectly spoken were all they achieved in six years' hard work. With hindsight, we can say the experiment was misguided: chimpanzees' voices are not man-like and are used only in emotional circumstances. Much more impressive is the recent success of Allen and Beatrice Gardner at Reno, in teaching sign language to their chimpanzee, Washoe.

Washoe was about a year old when, in the summer of 1966, she was put into a nursery. There she saw only specially trained humans who 'spoke' to her in American Sign Language, the hand-gesture language devised for the deaf. The Gardners used various devices for teaching Washoe to reply with the

Typical gestures used by humans and the chimpanzee Washoe in their exchanges. The first sign means 'more' and the second, with the finger drawn across the back of the hand, means 'tickle'. Washoe's vocabulary is mostly derived from the American Sign Language.

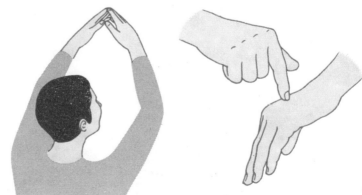

same gestures, including the use of rewards like tickling, which chimpanzees crave, but they found that taking the animal's hands and moving them through a gesture was particularly effective. Within two years, Washoe had a vocabulary of 34 signs. The animal showed no difficulty in generalising – from a particular flower, say, to the whole range of flowers, real or in pictures.

Washoe began spontaneously stringing signs together in meaningful combinations. No attempt had been made to encourage her to do so and, although her human companions did use combinations in addressing her, Washoe did not imitate them. 'Give me tickle' and 'listen eat' were typical invented utterances, the latter occurring when the alarm clock went off which signalled dinner-time. The chimpanzee coined her own term for the refrigerator: 'open food drink'. The Gardners reported in 1969, 'We believe now that it is the writers who would predict just what it is that no chimpanzee will ever do who must proceed with caution.'

Sayings of Sarah

David Premack takes the same view. As a psychologist at the University of California, Santa Barbara, he set out to communicate with his chimpanzee, Sarah, not to produce language-like operations for their own sake but in order to probe the

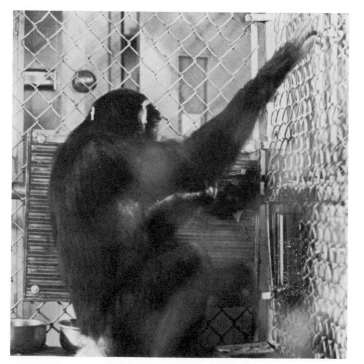

The chimpanzee Sarah in her cage with the vertical board on which she 'writes' with magnetised characters.

*Meanings of the first 34 **hand signs**
learnt by Washoe the chimpanzee:*

come	hear	flower	I
(= give me)	(= listen)	cover	(= me)
more	toothbrush	(= blanket)	shoes
up	drink	dog	smell
sweet	hurt	you	pants
open	sorry	napkin	clothes
tickle	funny	(= bib)	cat
go	please	in	key
out	food	brush	baby
hurry	(= eat)	hat	clean

An 18-month-old chimpanzee, Peony, is now at 'nursery school' in David Premack's group. She will learn similar skills.

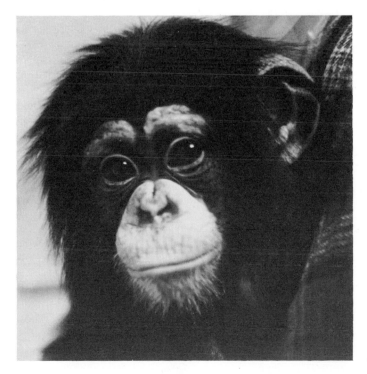

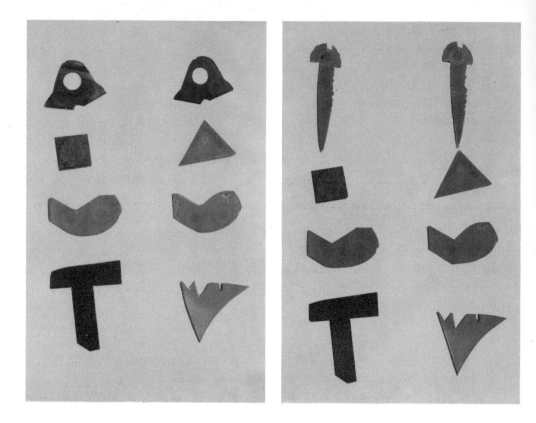

intellectual powers of the animal. Compared with Washoe, Sarah is said to use words in more elaborate logical operations.

Like the Gardners, Premack looked for a substitute for speech. He tried a machine in which an animal controlled the sounds it produced, but then he chose a method of reading and writing, using various coloured plastic shapes to represent words. The shapes contain magnetic material and cling to a vertical board. The use of written language allows the chimpanzee to study a question or a proposition which, if only spoken or gestured, might be forgotten before it had been analysed. The experimenter can also control the opportunity and scope of the chimpanzee to use the symbols, by restricting the supply; although one day Sarah stole the pieces and reportedly wrote out a question and answered it.

Sarah is older than Washoe; in 1970 when she was seven, she had been 'at school' for two years. She is less cosseted and in regular training sessions she learns by a stricter routine of trial and error, with rewards for successful performance. In this way she has slowly mastered about 130 words, and has also shown evidence of reasoning with them. Premack now suspects that chimpanzees have innate powers of language and that the learning process could be made much faster and less

Some of the magnetised symbols used for communicating with Sarah; they are read from top to bottom. On the left are two questions: '(Is it that) apple is red?' and '(Is it that) banana is yellow?'

On the right are the answers expected from Sarah; she replaces the first symbol in both columns by another symbol meaning 'yes'.

formal. Let me summarise what it is said that Sarah can do, before considering its credibility and its implications.

The following are English translations of some of the combinations of symbols with which Sarah can apparently cope, with a customary level of 80-per-cent proficiency:

1. *Sarah:* 'Mary give apple Sarah', the correct form for requesting food.
2. *Sarah:* 'Blue on green', as a description of the experimenter's arrangement of coloured cards.
3. *Experimenter:* 'Sarah insert banana pail apple dish', as an abridgement for 'Sarah insert banana pail; Sarah insert apple dish'.
4. *Experimenter:* 'What is (actual cork) to (another actual cork) – same or different?'
   Sarah: 'Same'.
5. *Experimenter:* 'Is (actual scissors) the same as (actual clothes peg) – yes or no?'
   Sarah: 'No'.
6. *Experimenter:* 'What is banana to (actual apple)?'
   Sarah: 'Not the name of', using one symbol which has that meaning.
7. *Experimenter:* 'Apple red banana yellow implies apple banana different colours – true or false?'
   Sarah: 'True'.

Premack remarked to me that the chimpanzee's attainment had confounded his original purpose. He wanted to find out what Sarah could not do – to mark out the limits of reasoning in the chimpanzee. In that way, he thought, he would help to show what was really special and unique about the mind of man. But as the tasks became more difficult, Sarah grew quicker to learn, not slower. There was nothing in sight that Sarah could not do. Premack would like to attempt the same kind of teaching and interrogation in species further from man.

To some of his colleagues, Premack's claims for Sarah are frankly incredible. Criticisms can be ventured at two levels: method and interpretation. The ghost of Clever Hans stalks through all animal-training experiments. Is it quite certain, for example, that no unconscious clues are being given to Sarah by the humans? To the visitor, Sarah seems to study the trainer more than the symbols on the board. Among the measures Premack has taken to check against that possibility is the use of strangers to interrogate Sarah. As for the interpretation of what Sarah does, the sternest question is whether the symbols are really words and sentences to her, or merely patterns to which she learns the correct response – as a more elaborate version of the learning by a rat to jump through a door with the appropriate markings.

Just because a human can assign verbal meanings to plastic shapes does not necessarily mean that the chimpanzee is thinking in anything like the same way. Premack has done careful tests to establish that the symbol for 'apple' really means apple to Sarah, but it may be rash at this stage to regard Sarah's apparent reasoning with symbols as entirely equivalent to human

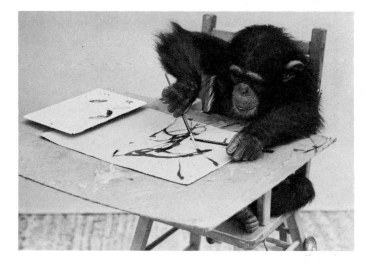

Chimpanzees have also been tested for their artistic ability and have shown some talent in fan-like paintings. (Congo at the London Zoo)

reasoning with words. Experts in language who have quizzed Premack intensively seem prepared to allow that something remarkable is going on, while hesitating to admit that it is language in the normal human sense.

The issue is wide open at the time of writing (1970). If we take Washoe and Sarah together, success in communicating with two different animals using very different methods gives mutual support to the experimenters. But it would be foolish not to remain cautious about their doings for the time being, because the implications are stupendous. Previous generations found that, contrary to all appearances, our earth is not the privileged hub of the universe and, worse still, we are descended from worms and apes. If chimpanzees really can reason with words in an abstract way, the shock to our human self-esteem will be in the same class.

The creative mind

Human beings are much more than talking machines in their creative activities. The explanatory problems posed by language are multiplied many times over, as much in everyday life as in the work of acknowledged geniuses. It is almost certainly

208

a misjudgement to focus attention on rare individuals and to suppose that the problem of explaining human achievements comes down to finding some peculiarity in the brains of Leonardo, Newton or Beethoven. One can allow that some individuals can alter history without separating them from the rest of us. Housewives who embellish their gossip with hyperbole and invention are using essentially the same brain mechanisms which Shakespeare used.

Contrasts in human creativity: the sanctified engineering of Chartres and (below) gossips who can rely as much on imagination as on mundane fact.

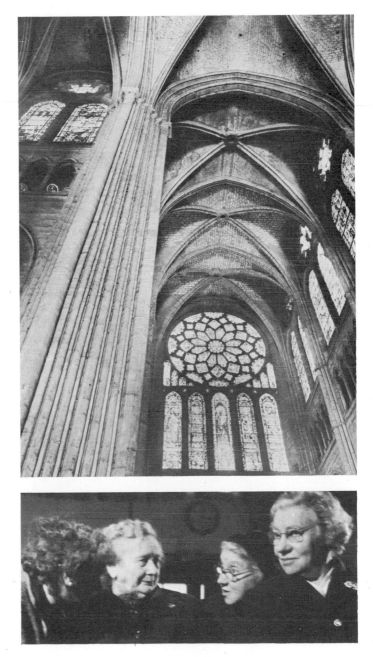

Although it is hard to relate to any particular function of the brain, the term 'intelligence' is supposed to denote a general ingredient in human ability. The mass schooling and complex citizen armies of our century have sustained a feudal urge to classify and grade everyone. Alfred Binet first devised intelligence testing for the French Ministry of Education, as a means of segregating the mentally deficient from normal classes; since then IQ tests have gained great importance in determining the education and careers of individuals. They have a certain success in predicting academic potential. But to say that there is much more to human mental powers than success in passing IQ tests or other examinations is no perverse opinion of my own.

During the past twenty years, psychologists dealing with children, and with adults in work where inventiveness is sought after, have paid increasing attention to 'divergent thinking' and 'creativity'. The IQ is primarily a measure of 'convergent thinking', roughly, the ability to learn or deduce correct answers to questions in contrast with 'divergent thinking', the ability to discover and invent. These different abilities may be found to a marked degree in the same talented

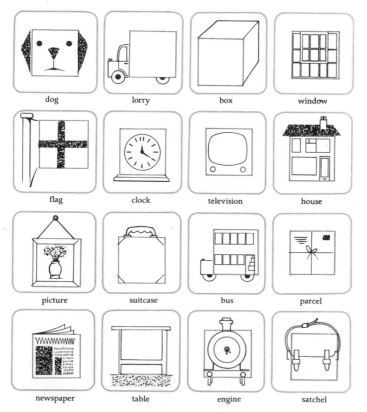

A typical creativity test: elaborate a square in as many ways as possible.

dog   lorry   box   window

flag   clock   television   house

picture   suitcase   bus   parcel

newspaper   table   engine   satchel

individual, but not necessarily so; many people with high IQs have scarcely a spark of originality in them.

Tests for creativity have been devised. They are less clear-cut than IQ tests, because there cannot be a correct answer planned in advance by the tester. Indeed, in a creativity test the 'right' or conventional answer is likely to be the wrong answer. A typical test is the Brick test – write down all the uses you can think of for a brick or, by drawing, elaborate a square in as many ways as possible.

About ten years ago, Jacob Getzels and Philip Jackson, with a team from the University of Chicago, carried out their famous inquiry into creativity among children at a private school. They picked out the two groups of children, 'High IQ' and 'High Creative'. One consisted of individuals scoring high in IQ tests (mean IQ 150) and relatively poorly in creativity tests, and the other of those whose IQ was markedly lower (mean IQ 127) but who did particularly well in creativity tests.

The investigators' first surprise came when they looked at the school achievement of the two groups, as measured by tests in English and mathematics: the High Creative group performed just as well as the High IQ group, despite the big difference in IQ. Such was the tyranny of the IQ test that, before this discovery, a child performing better at school than his IQ warranted was liable to be treated as a 'pusher', disliked by his teacher and perhaps even sent to a psychologist to find out what was wrong with him.

The High Creatives had a much greater sense of wit and humour than the High IQs; also a more frequent recourse to violence in their fantasies. Here is an account written, in an allotted time of four minutes, by one of Getzels and Jackson's High Creatives. It was in response to a picture of a man working late in the office:

> This man has just broken into this office of a new cereal company. He is a private eye employed by a competitor firm to find out the formula that makes the cereal bend, sag, and sway. After a thorough search of the office he comes upon what he thinks is the correct formula. He is now copying it. It turns out that it is the wrong formula and the competitor's factory blows up. Poetic justice!

The typical High IQ response to the same picture would dwell on the presumed hard work and ambition of the man in the office. Getzels and Jackson saw the High Creatives tending to free themselves from the stimulus given in the test, using it just as a point of departure, while the High IQs felt bound to the stimulus.

Refreshing though the fashionable interest in creativity may be, it usually deals with what kinds of people are the most creative, rather than with the inner processes involved. In any case, the spin-off of ideas, as tested in the examples given, is still only a first, primitive part of creative human thought and action. Dare we say anything, at this early stage of brain research, about the mechanisms underlying the work of a painter or a physicist? Did not Sigmund Freud say, apropos Dostoevsky: 'Before the problem of the creative artist analysis must, alas, lay down its arms'?

If we cannot even define the mental processes of high creative work, what hope is there of nailing them down to particular systems in the brain? None at all, if you want to know what brain cells were first fired with the concepts of St Peter's Basilica or the theory of universal gravitation. But to admit to complete bafflement would be to capitulate to mysticism. Let us insist, for a start, that brain cells and networks were responsible for those ideas. To say so is not to diminish the ideas, but rather to heighten our wonder that we, as assemblies of cells, are capable of them.

Machinery for judgement

The highest creative powers of man are plausibly rooted in brain mechanisms serving the most commonplace functions. We saw in Chapter 9 that the simplest processes of visual perception involve the formation of abstract 'models' in our

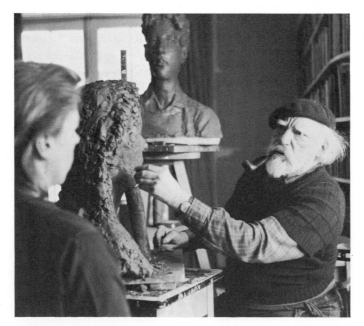

The artist uses his brain to modify reality with an imaginative vision. The late Augustus John at work.

minds, that the same machinery is used by the 'mind's eye', and that the raw material of the models can be reprocessed to produce completely new ideas, like the cobra in the bath. The dome of St Peter's presumably first appeared in the corresponding machinery inside Michelangelo's head. Similarly, the poet must use his hearing systems to imagine words and phrases. The experimental evidence that real perception interferes with imagination also suggests why isolation and absentmindedness are natural conditions for scientific and artistic work.

Genius is indeed close to madness and the flow of ideas in the head of a schizophrenic is an anguished form of invention. The fact that LSD and amphetamine produce crazy ideas and impressions by intervening in the transmissions between brain cells may persuade us that ideas do arise in the activity of those cells. But those artists who try to reinforce doubtful talents by taking such drugs might be better advised to try tranquillisers; after all, William Wordsworth traced the origin of poetry to 'emotion recollected in tranquillity'. The experiments which show that strain and excitement narrow attention to the chief task in hand fit nicely with the fact that ideas come so often when we are relaxed – in bed or in the bath.

Evidently the same brain mechanisms govern the scope of our attention to inward ideas as to external signals. Many are the instances of great creative workers waking up with a problem solved by unconscious operations. Usually this happens only when the individuals have expended months of conscious effort familiarising themselves with the problem; but not necessarily: Bertrand Russell said of the high point of his mathematical creativity, September 1900: 'Every evening the discussion ended with some difficulty and every morning I found that the difficulty of the previous evening had solved itself as I slept.'

> Tiger! Tiger! burning bright
> In the forests of the night,
> What immortal hand or eye
> Dare frame thy fearful symmetry?

William Blake's lines made the young Bertrand Russell faint when he first heard them. But, as John Cohen of Manchester University points out, the apparent simplicity of the lines is misleading. There are at least seven earlier drafts of the poem, so that Blake certainly did not hit on the words and their order at the first attempt; the mental search of the poet for his words does not involve only the unexplained mechanism and strategy for using the memory. There must also be a criterion for knowing when the search comes to an end, the point at which the poet, despairing of perfection, arrives at what he believes to be the best words in the best order. This means that he must have some idea of what he is looking for: somehow he is guided towards his goal. The strategy of this search will never be understood, in Cohen's judgement, until we have a psychology that takes account of information generated within the brain as well as the objectively specifiable information coming from outside.

In any case, the flow of original ideas is plainly not enough. Critical judgement and the selection of a good idea out of the mass of bad ideas thrown up by the active imagination are what distinguish the sane creative worker from the madman. But judgement, too, is involved in relatively low-level functions of the brain – for example, in recognising a friend from a distance by his gait or in spotting the rotten apple in a heap of good ones. To say so certainly does not explain judgement but at least we allot such mundane tasks to brain systems, animal as well as human. We can invoke the same processes for higher purposes.

Our hunting forefathers who suddenly spotted a deer half-hidden among the trees felt a 'thump', the excitement of recognition, from some coupling between the visual model-making sites in the brain, the deep-lying emotional sites and probably other regions as well. We may imagine that the aesthetic judgement of rightness or 'truth', produced by a painting or a mathematical equation, is rooted in the same brain systems. The subjective reality of the lusty pursuit of the satisfaction of a good idea appears in the accompanying testimony of Richard Feynman, a Nobel-prizewinning American, and one of the acknowledged masters of theoretical physics of our time.

The physical realities of the appropriate systems are adumbrated, at least, by judgement-like responses to electrical stimulation during brain operations, especially low in the side of the roof of the brain – Penfield's 'interpretive cortex'. Patients report the experience of *déjà vu* ('I've been here before') or the converse feeling that everything is absurd. Such feelings certainly seem to operate in aesthetic appreciation. A cynic has said that a prudent artist produces the same kind of work repeatedly, on the principle that we like what we know, because we can feel like connoisseurs.

Laughter is another unmistakable mechanism of judgement. A customary topic for those who worry about how the body and the conscious mind interact is how physical pain can so afflict the mind; it seems to me equally appropriate to ask how

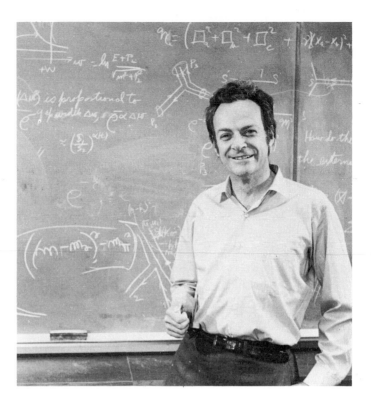

Richard Feynman, an outstanding theoretical physicist. When he was asked to describe the inner experiences of a discoverer, he responded in his forthright way with the comments given below.

Sometimes I feel like an ape, trying to figure out how nature's going to behave, fooling around with all those symbols. I've always thought about what it is that goes on when I think about these things. I realise it's a big mix of pictures and symbols, and in my head there's a kind of confusing mess. But the symbols are inventions of other people which make our thinking about nature efficient. So I've got a great advantage over the apes, because I have the experience of all the other individuals who've invented these things to help me to think. And I've invented something, too, called the Feynman diagram, that other people use. It helps them to analyse the way nature's going to behave.

My father got me interested in all these things by telling me how wonderful nature was. But he couldn't know the terrible excitement of making a new discovery. You get so excited you can't calculate, you can't think any more. It isn't just that nature's wonderful because if someone tells me the answer to a problem I'm working on, it's nowhere near as exciting as if I work it out myself.

a passing thought can make the body shake, the breathing become explosive, and the tears flow happily. But learned ponderosity on the subject of humour is itself laughable, reminiscent of the story of how the philosopher Immanuel Kant finally plucked up courage to call on a lady to propose marriage, only to find that she had left the district twenty years before. Jokes, too, desert you when you stop to think too hard about them, for they are typically instantaneous in their effect. Yet the sages are quite right: humour is no laughing matter.

Those feelings of absurdity produced by electrical stimulation of the temporal lobe probably help to locate one of the brain mechanisms involved, but absurdity can evoke anger instead of laughter. The 'laughter site' in the brain was discovered accidently by a distinguished German surgeon, Richard Hassler, during an operation in 1955, and confirmed on subsequent occasions.

It is a region of the thalamus, deep inside the brain, where stimulation can make the most gravely ill or anxious patient smile or laugh out loud. Many signalling systems of brain and body converge at the thalamus, so there is plenty of scope for

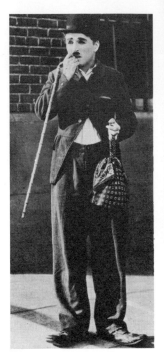

An art that tickles the very centre of the brain. (Chaplin in Modern Times)

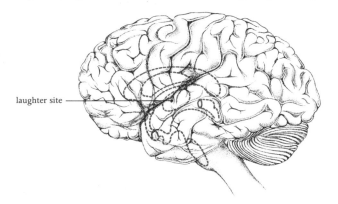

laughter site

a pooling of influences, so far untraced, to turn a tickle, a surprise or a witticism into a tightening of the diaphragm or an outright laugh.

The sceptical reader will see that we have clutched at experimental straws in our search for a basis of creativity in brain mechanisms. Ulric Neisser, introducing his recent book, *Cognitive Psychology*, apologises for devoting so little space to thinking, concept-formation and the like. 'It is because I believe there is still relatively little to say about them, even after 100 years of psychological research.' For my part, I have skirted a great deal of inconclusive experiment and theory in aesthetics. The most persuasive story relating human intellectual powers to the brain is that of their gradual emergence as the brain grows during childhood.

216

A contemporary poet's view of the creative process comes impressively close to the psychological idea of brain-made 'models' of the world.

A WAY OF LOOKING

It is the association after all
We seek, we would retrace our thoughts to find
The thought of which this landscape is the image,
Then pay the thought and not the landscape homage.
It is as if the tree and waterfall
Had their first roots and source within the mind.

But something plays a trick upon the scene:
A different kind of light, a stranger colour
Flows down on the appropriated view.
Nothing within the mind fits. This is new.
Thought and reflection must begin again
To fit the image and to make it true.

Elizabeth Jennings

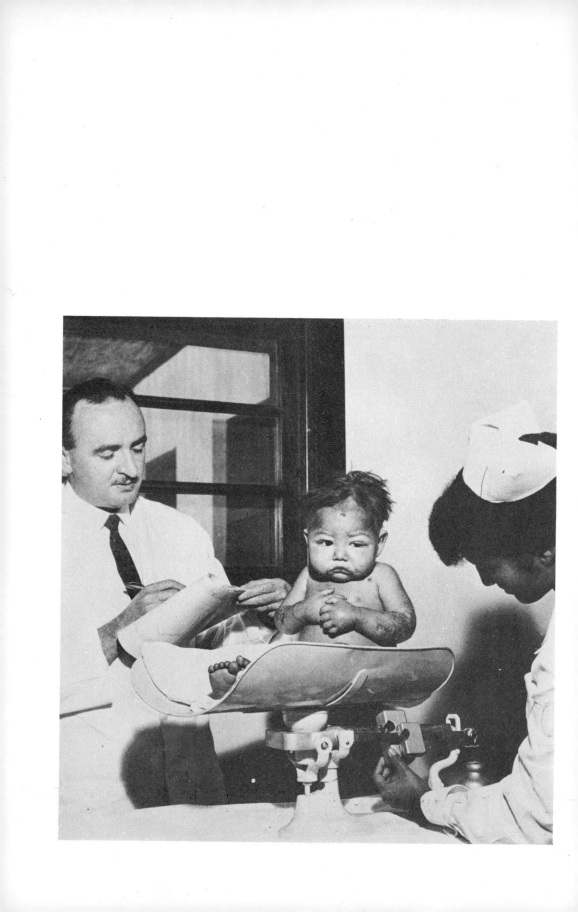

12   Making and Marring

The growing brain prepares itself for particular events to occur at critical periods. Provided they do occur, the child will progress to new accomplishments. While the contributions of heredity and upbringing to human variations are still debated, malnutrition is imposing a tax on human mental powers.

A Latin-American child suffering from severe protein malnutrition, with the characteristic sad expression of the kwashiorkor victim

A bright orange flashing light is the first thing that chicks see after they hatch in a laboratory at Madingley, near Cambridge. A group of them, born into darkness, are put in individual cages around the lamp. Before long, each of them becomes fascinated by the light and nestles up against the side of the cage nearest to it. This is not just curiosity. The chicks take the light to be their mother, because it is the most conspicuous object in their young lives. In later tests the chick will run towards a similar flashing lamp, even under trying conditions.

'Imprinting' is the name given by Konrad Lorenz to this special learning mechanism. It makes early visual experience particularly forceful in its effect on the chicks' subsequent conduct. When humans intervene at hatching they can imprint the chicks with bizarre substitutes – a toy, a cardboard box, the experimenter himself. Thereafter, a chick will run to, or follow, his pseudo-mother just as faithfully as he would tag on to the real hen.

In the experiments at Madingley, Gregory Bateson and Gabriel Horn of Cambridge University collaborated with Steven Rose, from Britain's new Open University, to look for specific chemical changes in the chicks' brains during imprinting. Holger Hydén in Göteborg detected the manufacture of specific chemical materials, RNA and protein (see page 121), in the brains of rats learning to use their 'weak' hands. The three British researchers reported similar changes in imprinted chicks. More newly-made RNA and protein are found, in parts of their brains, than in corresponding parts in chicks which have missed the imprinting experience.

Imprinting is one of the most important events in a young bird's life. It can only happen once, and that during the first 24 hours out of the egg. There is a period of an hour or so, a few hours after hatching, when imprinting occurs most strongly. So critical is the timing that, if a bird hatches exceptionally late, it may miss the opportunity altogether. The capacity for imprinting has been built by evolution into many animal species where the young are mobile at birth and there would otherwise be a risk of them wandering away from their mothers. It occurs in sheep and probably explains Mary of the nursery rhyme as a pseudo-mother:

> And everywhere that Mary went,
> That lamb was sure to go.

Nothing quite as theatrical as imprinting occurs in human babies in the normal course of development. We have plenty of time to identify our mothers before we become physically able to desert them. But imprinting is just an extreme instance of a general policy of nature, from which humans are not excluded. It is that the development of a particular mental faculty often depends upon a coincidence. The brain must be ripe and the appropriate event must occur in the environment.

Experiments on vision in animals supply some direct proof of critically-timed environmental effects on the connections in the brain. David Hubel and Torsten Wiesel, at the Harvard Medical School, find that a kitten's brain, at birth, possesses the elaborate system of detectors of lines and patterns, ready to work. But if one eye is kept closed for as little as four days, during the second month of the kitten's life, the system of detectors in the brain, corresponding to that eye, ceases to function and it does not recover. Plainly, there is a critical period when the visual system is maturing and use of the eye is essential if powers that already exist are to be reconfirmed.

Biologists who watch unrestrained animals, to see how they behave, call themselves ethologists. They are inclined to scoff at the vast number of laboratory experiments which use pent-up animals to test psychological theories. Too little attention is paid, they say, to the complex ways in which animals conduct themselves naturally. From their careful observations of animals in free-ranging conditions, ethologists are led to talk of innate mechanisms in the brains of animals, which have to be triggered or confirmed in operation by events in the environment. Recognition of particular signals provides some examples. Young gulls will beg for food when they see markings like those carried by adult gulls on their heads.

Similar mechanisms exist in the brains of young monkeys. Gene Sackett of the University of Wisconsin has taken the lessons of the ethologists seriously. He demonstrated inborn recognition of special signals by separating baby monkeys from their mothers when they were less than a day old, so that they could not be taught. He reared them individually in cages where they could see no other monkeys. When they were two weeks old, the young monkeys began to see photographic slides of monkeys projected on to one wall of each cage; after they were four months old they saw movies as well. Sackett observed the responses of the young monkeys to pictures of different kinds.

A picture of an infant monkey or a picture of an adult monkey making a threatening gesture provoked the most excitement in the young viewer – exploration, climbing, calling, play movements and so on. Other slides of monkeys had much less effect. Remember, these young monkeys had never seen live monkeys, nor had they any chance to learn the meaning of these appearances. Nevertheless their responses were unmistakable. What was even more interesting, a threat produced no sign of fear or disturbance in the young monkeys until they were about $2\frac{1}{2}$ months old. Then they suddenly began to be very fearful of the threat slides, which they had enjoyed many times before. Sackett believes that an innate brain mechanism must be maturing at that age, which 'tells' the young monkey that the threatening pose of another monkey means danger. But later the fear wore off, presumably because no real danger materialised.

Although comparable experiments in humans are out of the question, harmless tests in very young babies have shown that the human brain is prewired at birth to respond to human faces and human voices, in preference to other sights and sounds. Evidence accumulates for a sketchy biography written in the genes of each one of us. It does not, of course, foretell the detailed stories of our lives. It provides that definite events become due at particular periods when our brains are ripe for certain crucial kinds of interaction with the environment, and particular stages in our development are reached. Shakespeare descanted on seven ages of man, but most of the 'ages' of man's brain are reached and passed in childhood.

Birth of the brain

As his big head suggests, the brain grows faster than the child in the earliest years of life. When the new human being begins to develop from the little round speck of the fertilised egg, the first clear signs of the knobs that will become the brain appear about three weeks after conception, when the embryo is only about three millimetres long. By the time the baby is born, his brain weighs about one-quarter of the adult brain weight, although his body is only one-twentieth of its adult weight. At birth, the brain already possesses virtually its whole complement of electrical brain cells, the neurons. But the brain is still growing quickly at that time, doubling in weight within the first six months after birth; when the child is five, his brain will be 90 per cent of its full adult weight.

The discovery of two distinct 'growth spurts', when cells multiply most rapidly in the young human brain, was announced in 1970 by John Dobbing and Jean Sands of Manchester University. They took the amount of genetic material (DNA) in the brain of the embryo as a measure of the number of cells. They found it increased very rapidly in the period fifteen to twenty weeks after conception. Dobbing and Sands think that this is the period when most of the neurons of the brain are first formed. At about 25 weeks, a new phase of cell multiplication begins, not quite so intensive as the first, but continuing right through the time of birth and for more than a year thereafter. They take the view that most of the cells being formed in this second period are the ancillary glue cells (glia) rather than neurons.

In some animals, new neurons form even after birth, though it is unlikely that many do so in humans. Joseph Altman of the

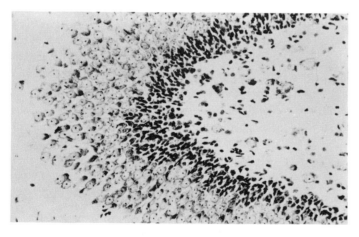

Some new neurons form after birth, according to Joseph Altman. In a section of the brain of a 30-day-old kitten, a stain distinguishes between the pale neurons already formed and a layer of darker, newly-forming neurons.

Right: How the visible connections between neurons develop in the human infant after birth is shown by tracings from the same region at the side of the brain: right, at 3 months; far right, at 24 months. (After Conel)

Massachusetts Institute of Technology injected into new-born rats a radioactive material which is incorporated in the genetic material of cells which are dividing. In a series of such experiments in the 1960s he showed that not only glue cells but also small neurons were being formed for some time after birth in important regions of the rats' brains. Even in young adults the formation of these new cells did not cease altogether.

Although a human baby possesses virtually all his neurons at birth, that does not mean that the brain is ready to work. It is more like a kit of parts than a finished machine. The neurons

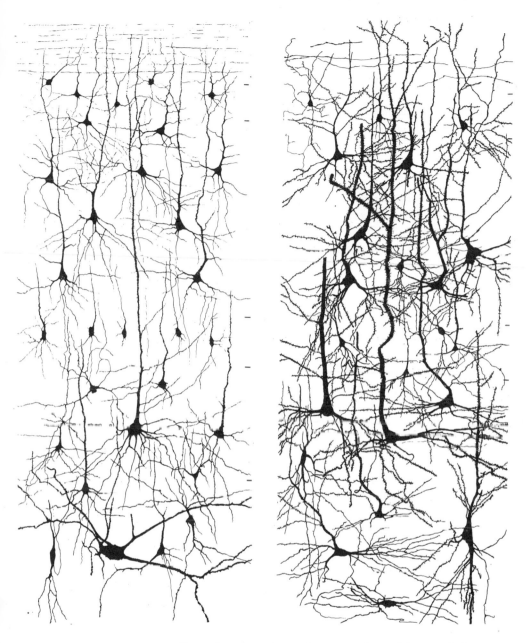

themselves have to continue growing, taking up their proper positions and making vast numbers of new connections with one another. And the newly-forming glue cells are not mere space-fillers – they are essential for the efficient working of the brain.

Growth is not uniform throughout the brain during the formative years and some regions 'ripen' long before others. In the very young human embryo, the brain stem is the first part to develop. The roof of the brain, the cerebral cortex, begins to grow in earnest about ten weeks after conception.

The cerebellum, the 'little brain' concerned with balance and skilled movements, does not start growing rapidly until shortly before birth, but it continues to do so for about a year after birth.

Within a given region of the brain, there is immense variation in the state of development. As the accompanying diagram of the cerebral cortex shows, the upper central and hindmost regions, concerned with bodily sensation, control of movement, hearing and vision, mature early. The front and lower sides mature later. That, too, is an oversimplification. Within the motor strip, for example, the parts controlling trunk and arm movements are in advance of other parts controlling leg and finger movements.

A baby prematurely born is almost oblivious of its surroundings except that bright light or loud noises can produce some primitive reactions, which do not correspond to 'seeing' or 'hearing' in the normal sense. Even if he is born three months early, he has to wait until that period has elapsed before he begins to show the responses to lights and sounds

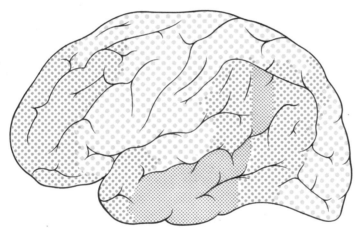

The whole brain does not mature at the same time; the deeply coloured areas are last to mature. Below: how the width of one layer in the front of a child's brain increases after birth. (After Vogt and Polyakov)

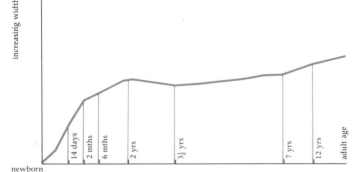

characteristic of a baby born at the right time. In other words, powers develop when the brain is ready, and not before.

Judging by the immature state of the cerebral cortex, it may play very little part in the life of the child at the time of birth. He may be completely dependent upon the inner regions of the brain. Even the motor strip is not active at birth. Not until the child is about three months old does the roof of the brain begin to intervene in earnest in the control of movements of the arms, with the first signs of co-ordination of hand and eye.

The peculiar calendar

The purposeful grasp of the baby's hand emerges quite slowly from the display of mindless reflexes and their subsequent mastery. Thomas Twitchell of the Massachusetts Institute of Technology has studied this development in detail. The pulling action of the arms is at first simply a response to a stretching of the muscles. At about two weeks after birth an object touching the palm of the hand can evoke it. After another two weeks,

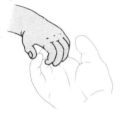

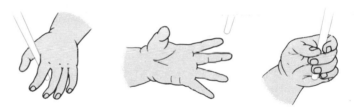

A baby develops the power to grasp. After the 'grasp reflex' (left) is fully formed, an 'instinctive grasp reaction' gradually matures, by way of an orienting response and a grasping action, to a fully developed grasp.

thumb and index finger will begin a grasping action. By about three months this grasp reflex is fully developed, using all fingers first to grab the object and then to cling on to it.

Then another phase of development begins – the instinctive grasp reaction. Gradually, during the following months, the hand will begin to twist, grope and reach out, in pursuit of any object touching it. The eyes are not involved, nor is it an entirely reliable movement; contact with the object on certain parts of the hand will produce a withdrawal reflex. But the child is now ready to convert the primitive grasps into purposeful movements with co-ordination of hand and eye.

A fascinating stage around seven months is worth mentioning, when a child uses his eyes to aim his hand at the object of interest but closes his eyes as he launches his hand to grasp it. Evidently he does so to cut out information he has not yet learned to employ properly. The automatic grasping actions can still be quite easily evoked at the age of five. Some adults with brain damage will revert to these automatic grasping 225 responses of babyhood. They occur particularly in cases of damage towards the front of the brain.

A baby is much more 'subhuman' in his mental powers than many mothers may realise. Throughout the first years of life, the child progresses as various parts of the brain mature and come into service. A new-born baby will make automatic walking movements with his legs when held upright, but he will not learn to walk until essential parts of the brain are ready – in the motor strip, the cerebellum and elsewhere – and switch on. Indeed, 'learning to walk' is a somewhat misleading way of describing the event, though practice is obviously involved. The baby does not learn to walk at will, in the way that an older child learns to skate or ride a bicycle. When his brain is ready, he walks.

And when his brain is ready, he will talk. The powers of speech also develop in a predictable manner according to a timetable, in close synchronism with advances in walking, jumping and so on. Provided a child hears language used in the normal way – in what Eric Lenneberg calls 'simple immersion in the sea of language' – he will pass steadily from one level of comprehension and utterance to the next. From the first forming of consonants at around six months he will progress to mastery of colloquial grammar by the age of three. If deafness or other disorders delay the acquisition of language, or if brain injuries in early life destroy language already acquired, a child can still make excellent progress, up to the age of about 10; after that, the difficulties become greater.

Up to the same age, too, children can learn foreign languages in a non-academic way, much as they learn their native language. But in the early teens, as the brain finally matures, it switches off its powers of spontaneous language acquisition. Thereafter language is no longer in the gift of nature but becomes a matter of toiling over textbooks. Wilder Penfield, who lives in the bilingual province of Quebec, has for long urged educators to take account of the 'peculiar calendar' of the human mind and to ensure that every child learns both English and French before the age of 10.

A wise mother may know the effect of immaturity and try to avoid telling a two-year-old child to stop doing something, because she is likely to prompt him to do it more energetically than ever. The slowly-maturing frontal lobes seem to be required for a child to respond correctly to verbal instructions. Without any perversity on the part of the child, the immaturity of his brain may make it physically impossible not to *do* what he is told *not* to do. Alexander Luria of Moscow

has summed up this effect and others, in pointing out their

close correspondence with abnormal performance in adults with damage to the frontal lobes. Some examples of typical reactions of young children are shown in the table below.

Until the front of the brain is well developed, a child is incapable of obeying some verbal instructions. (Data from Alexander Luria)

Age of child (approximate, years: months)	Objects available	Adult's instruction	Child's action
1:3	Toy rabbit and hen	(a) 'Give me the rabbit' (repeated several times)	Offers rabbit
		(b) 'Give me the hen'	Offers rabbit
2:0	Box, cup, hidden penny	(a) 'The penny is under the cup; give me the penny' (repeated several times)	Lifts cup
		(b) 'The penny is under the box; give me the penny'	Lifts cup
2:0	Rubber bulb and recorder	(a) 'Press the ball'	Presses
		(b) 'Don't press any more'	Presses harder
2:3	Rubber bulb and recorder; lamp	(a) 'When you see the light you must press the ball'	Presses at once
		(b) (Light comes on)	Stops pressing
2:6	Rubber bulb and recorder; coloured lamps	(a) 'When you see the green light say "go" and press the ball'	Presses at once
		(b) (Green light comes on)	Says 'go' and stops pressing
3:3	As before	(a) As before, plus 'When you see the red light say "no" and stop pressing the ball'	Waits
		(b) (Green light comes on)	Says 'go' and presses
		(c) (Red light comes on)	Says 'no' and presses harder

The young child understands the instructions perfectly well; whenever necessary, subsidiary tests confirm that. His brain is simply unable to act on them. As Luria comments, the development of the highest forms of conscious, self-regulated activity is by no means a simple process. Not until the child is four years old or more is his brain ready to learn to carry out a complex programme of actions deliberately, in accordance with unrepeated verbal instructions.

The involvement of the frontal lobes is vividly demonstrated when an adult with damage to the front of the brain responds to verbal commands like a two-year-old. The patient often perseveres in an action after he has been told to stop or to do something else. Here is one of Luria's frontal-lobe patients drawing figures by instruction.

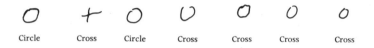

| Circle | Cross | Circle | Cross | Cross | Cross | Cross |

Maturing intellect

Psychologists have known for a long time that the way a child sets about looking for a missing object is a useful indicator of his level of mental development. In John Cohen's group at Manchester, the child's ability to search systematically for a hidden object is examined with an automatic machine. He is presented with a square array of 144 holes and told that one

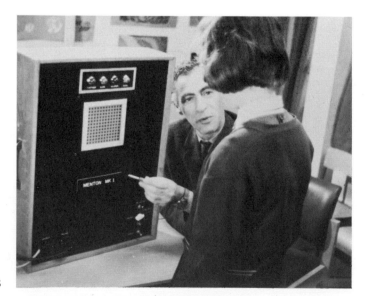

The 'hidden treasure' game at the University of Manchester. The older child is much more logical than a younger child in using the signal lights to help her find the hole that marks the treasure.

Right: Jean Piaget of Geneva.

of them represents hidden treasure. He can shift a peg one move at a time to look for it and coloured lights (green, red and amber) tell him whether the move takes him nearer or farther away or makes no difference.

The older a child is, the more information he will derive from the hints given from the lights. An eight-year-old will stab rather wildly at the board, just hoping to guess the best move; as a result his path wanders erratically over the board and it takes him a long time to find the treasure. A thirteen-year-old, on the other hand, will get there much faster and more logically and with greater confidence in his judgement.

That we have charts of the stages of a child's intellectual progress is mainly due to Jean Piaget of Geneva University. In nearly half a century of work he has made many comparisons between the mind of the child and the mind of the adult, and between children of different ages. On its basis he has built a theory of thinking, which is his expression of the logic of mental operations; but we shall leave that aside to concentrate on the stages of development distinguished by Piaget. There are five stages, and I must emphasise that the ages given are merely typical. The tags given to the phrases are less formal than Piaget's own (in brackets), just as the notes are a gross simplification of what he says about them.

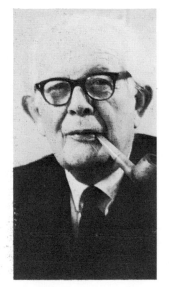

1. *Grab and search* (sensory-motor period, 0 – 2 years). The baby cannot carry out internalised mental operations in the adult sense. He will, however, learn to pull a rug to reach an object, or to move a pillow to find an object. He comes to realise that objects endure when they are out of sight.

2. *Learning symbols* (pre-operative thought, 2 – 4 years). In this period the child is learning to talk and, more generally, he is learning that actions can be imitated and that a symbol can represent an object or event. There is no clear distinction between thought and reality, or between living and inanimate objects.

3. *Fixed judgement* (intuitive thought, 4 – 7 years). Now we have Piaget's famous test with beads in jars. A child in this phase has advanced in other respects but, if one of two equal jars of beads is emptied into a thinner jar, the child cannot believe that the number of beads remains the same; either there are fewer because the jar is thinner, or more because the column is taller.

4. *Common sense* (concrete operations, 8 – 11 years). At around the age of 7 or 8, the material world at last begins to make sense, with the categories, positions and relationships of

objects in space and time well understood. But the child has to have concrete objects in front of him to be able to deal with them coherently. And, even then, 'common sense' can mislead him into supposing, for example, that a remodelled lump of clay has changed its volume with the change in shape.

5. *Abstract thought* (propositional operations, 11 – 14 years). *Homo sapiens* begins to live up to his name in this adolescent phase. He can reason with statements about events as well as with the events themselves. The intellectual skills collected during childhood are merged together in a fine logical apparatus which can deal with hypothetical ideas as well as with actuality.

Does intellectual development in later childhood depend upon the maturing of further particular brain systems? To assert that this is so, we have to rely at present on circumstantial evidence and on the close analogy with the earlier stages. There are abstract concepts which a child simply cannot understand until he attains a certain mental age, no matter how bright he is. And just as learning to reach out and grasp a physical object occurred in a well-defined sequence of stages, with the development of the brain after birth, so there is an orderly advancement in the grasping of ideas, during the first 11 years of life.

With no definite disclosures yet coming from brain research, there are plausible suggestions that new interconnections have to form between different regions of the brain if the child is to pass from one of these later intellectual stages to the next. We can be sure that the brain is not completely formed at least until the important changes in sexuality have exerted their physical effects at puberty.

Effects of upbringing

A startling if not shocking effect of a baby's environment on his development turned up in the early 1960s. Burton White and Richard Held of the Massachusetts Institute of Technology studied conditions in a hospital caring for unwanted newborn children. For their first four months the babies lay in plain cribs – 'a bland and uniform world', was how White and Held described it. The investigators obtained permission to try enriching the visual world of some of the children, by equipping their cribs with coloured sheets and hanging a collection of gaily-coloured objects over their heads. The babies so treated developed their ability to make purposeful reaching

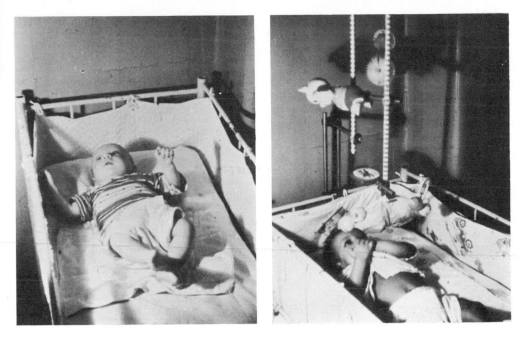

Unwanted babies were found living in a visual desert (above). Giving them something to look at (right) greatly accelerated their development.

movements with their hands nearly seven weeks earlier than did the children in the standard cribs – and this during a period of life when advances in performance from one month to the next are very rapid indeed.

Experiments on the upbringing of animals can look deeper, at physical consequences in the brain. Does the experience of a rat have any detectable effect on the structure of his brain? A team that has attacked this problem consists of a psychologist, Mark Rosenzweig, a biochemist, Edward Bennett, and an anatomist, Marian Diamond. In their experiments at the University of California, Berkeley, from 1959 onwards, the answer turned out to be far from obscure.

For 'enriched' experience, rats were put in groups of 10 or 12 into big cages, with plenty of toys, swings, ladders and the like, to interest them. Litter-mates of these animals went into individual cages with ample food but nothing much to do. The rats reared in the 'enriched' environment grew bigger brains than those of animals kept in the standard conditions of the laboratory colony, which in turn showed bigger brains than the rats from the 'impoverished' environment.

Overall, there was about 5 per cent difference in weight for the cerebral cortex. When the regions at the back of the brain are singled out for comparison, in rats from the enriched and impoverished cages, the difference in weight is up to about 10 per cent. The cortex of the privileged rats is visibly thicker, the cell bodies of the individual neurons are larger and the number of glue cells (glia) is markedly greater. Certain 231 materials, enzymes involved in the chemical transmission systems between neurons, are more abundant.

In the earliest experiments, rats spent 80 days continuously in the enriched environment. Two hours a day for 30 days in the 'play-cage' now turns out to be sufficient to produce pronounced changes in the brain. But the success of these experiments at Berkeley has become tantalising, because they are difficult to interpret. No one has yet convincingly related these physical differences to lasting differences in the learning and reasoning powers of the rats from the different environments. The Berkeley group has found that rats from the enriched environment are superior in problem-solving in certain tests, but the scores of enriched and impoverished tend to converge as testing is continued. Furthermore, some tests show differences only at certain ages, whereas others uniformly show the enriched rats to be superior, and the complexity of such testing should not be underestimated.

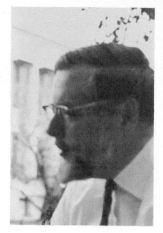

Mark R. Rosenzweig.

In this connection, Harry Harlow's experiments (see p. 34) in which young monkeys were kept in isolation much like that of the impoverished rats of Berkeley showed quite firmly that, however much emotional damage the monkeys had suffered, their ultimate intellectual performance was indistinguishable from that of more favoured monkeys – at any rate after long pre-training.

The Berkeley investigators have now turned to another question. Even the enriched cages of their rats may be a poor substitute for the life of young rats in the wild; they may represent 'less impoverished' rather than truly enriched conditions. To find a more natural baseline, Rosenzweig and his colleagues have begun trapping wild deer-mice in the Berkeley area and comparing their brains on capture with the effects of various artificial modes of life.

There are other grounds than brain enlargement for supposing that an interesting environment is better than a dull one for developing young minds. If we take the simple-minded view that big brains are better than small ones, do the Berkeley experiments tell us anything about the ingredients of an interesting environment? Nothing directly about human children, obviously; but what may be significant is that the circumstances producing brain enlargement in rats seem to be remarkably specific. David Krech, who was an early participant in the experiments, emphasises this point.

Several kinds of experience afforded to the rats by Rosenzweig and his collaborators produced little or no increase in the brain size. Physical exercise, varied visual

stimulation, fondling, the company of a brother rat, learning to

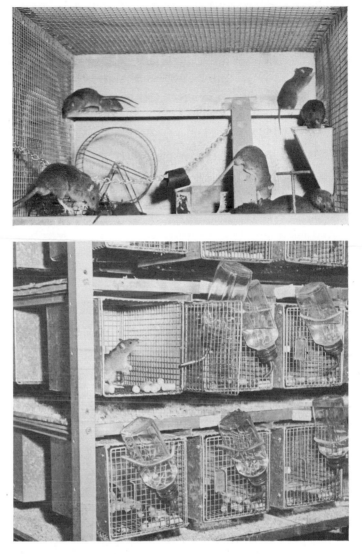

Enriched environment. At Berkeley, rats enjoy a 'University of California education' with a variety of objects to stimulate them.

Impoverished environment. Single rats live in cages with solid walls (a door has been opened to show one animal).

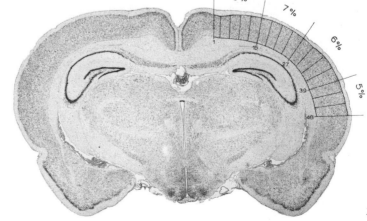

A section of a rat's cerebral cortex towards the back of the brain. The percentages shown represent the differences in the thickness of the cortex at various positions, between 'enriched' and 'impoverished' rats, after two to three months in their respective conditions. Statistically the results are very reliable; 100 animals were used in this particular comparison.

6%   7%   6%   5%

press levers for food – none of these was effective. Only freedom to roam around a large, object-filled space produced substantial changes. Krech suggests that for each species of animal there are specific experiences which are maximally efficient in developing the brain: he mocks the 'educators who would bombard the child from infancy on with every kind of stimulus change imaginable'. His own guess is that, for humans, the most important experiences are those of language.

Nature and nurture

The hottest political issue in psychology and brain research is stirred and restirred by discoveries of the kind just described. When I say political I mean precisely that. The Second World War flowed from the proposition that one nation was genetically superior to others and questions of race remain prominent today. The recent Chinese Cultural Revolution, by contrast, was waged in the conviction that a farm worker is potentially as capable as a professor. Trotsky once summed up the communist belief in the perfectibility of man by saying that the average human being would be raised to the level of Aristotle, Goethe and Marx.

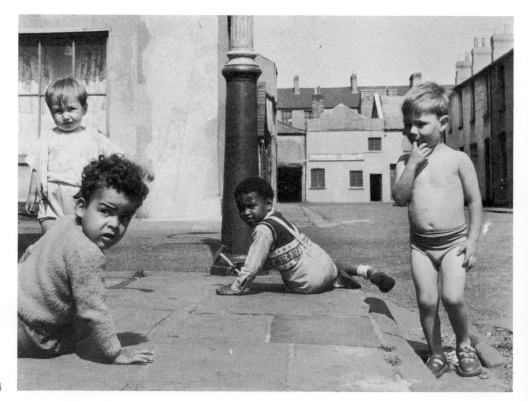

The question that is so ancient and yet so topical is 'nature versus nurture'. To what extent is heredity responsible for the variations between individuals and to what extent are they determined by the environment in which they grow up?

Gross genetic defects are known which are plainly linked with effects on intellect, social conduct and mental health. One is PKU, phenylketonuria, a metabolic defect causing brain damage and feeblemindedness unless detected at birth and treated with special diets. Among convicts there is a disproportionate number of very tall men and among these another blatant genetic abnormality occurs remarkably often. Most human beings have 46 chromosomes, which are the vehicles of the genes present in most cells of the body. Some of the convicts have the wrong number, being most commonly burdened by an additional Y (male) chromosome.

Before accepting such facts as proof of the overriding impor tance of heredity in the brain we have to ask a question which cannot yet be answered. Are these congenital conditions with effects on intellect and conduct so atypical that the individuals should be separated from the argument, just as you would exclude thalidomide babies from a discussion of the inheritance of athletic powers? Or does the whole population carry a burden of bad genes affecting intellect and conduct, genes

Contrasts in environments: a playground in Accra, Ghana, equipped by the United Nations Children's Fund (UNICEF) and (left) children in Cardiff. A close comparison with the Berkeley rats should not be drawn.

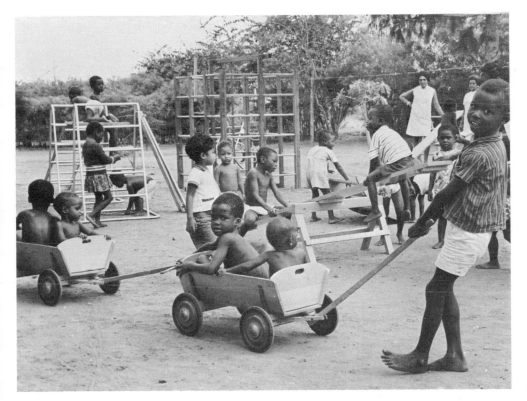

less conspicuous in their effects but nevertheless producing a wide range of ability and self-control?

Schizophrenia and related milder (schizoid) disorders seem now, after half a century of argument, to be established as hereditary diseases. Schizophrenia may be due to a single 'bad' gene while other genes are able to moderate its effect in schizoidia. Leonard Heston of the University of Iowa estimates that four people in every hundred are affected by the disease to some extent. The argument which delayed this conclusion was of the classic kind. The evidence was clear enough: children of schizophrenic parents were much more likely than other children to be schizophrenic themselves. But the treatment they received was very possibly responsible. Even now, no one would dispute the effect of environment in exaggerating or moderating the effects of heredity. The disentanglement of this hoary issue gives hope that other complex nature-nurture issues will be resolved.

The nature-nurture controversy, perennial in public affairs, flowers vividly every few years in academic circles. In 1969, Arthur Jensen, of the University of California, Berkeley, brought it to life with a lengthy report on IQ scores. His conclusion, which did not go unremarked in political circles, was that American negroes were on average less 'intelligent' than American whites, by 15 points on the IQ scale. There is no longer much dispute about the evidence that American negroes do, on average, score comparatively poorly in IQ tests, but the argument about why they should do so continues fiercely.

The test questions may be culturally biased in favour of whites and the well-to-do, or the negroes may be poorly motivated to do well in the tests. Even if the tests are realistic, to conclude that negroes score poorly because of racial heredity depends on assumptions about nature, nurture and their interaction which are beyond the present competence of science to verify. Critics who have varied Jensen's assumptions slightly have been able to account for virtually the whole of the IQ score difference as an environmental effect.

Identical twins separated at birth are much sought after by psychologists anxious to determine the relative importance of nature and nurture. Identical twins are genetically identical and tend to be very similar in intellectual performance when reared together. As they also receive identical treatment in such circumstances, that by itself would say nothing about the issue, if it were not for the fact that fraternal twins show marked differences in IQ scores. Identical twins usually persist in showing similar IQ scores when reared separately, which testifies to the great influence of heredity; yet occasionally one identical twin turns out to score much higher than the other, which testifies to the great influence of environment.

Daniel Bovet, of Sassari University in Italy, has set out, quite explicitly, to test nature versus nurture in different strains of mice. In laboratory strains of animals, selective breeding can reduce almost to vanishing point the variations between individuals within the strain, so that they are like a population of identical twins. And the chosen characteristic can be a particular level of performance in a particular laboratory test. Bovet has mice which perform consistently well in a 'shuttle-box', and another strain which does consistently badly. In this apparatus, a mouse has to learn to move smartly through a small opening to the other end of the box when a light comes on, in order to avoid an electric shock.

By the mid-1960s, Bovet and his colleagues had these two strains of mice whose marked differences in learning ability they thoroughly understood. For their nature-nurture experiment, the mice were switched for weaning: the young of poor learners were reared by good learner mothers, and vice versa. When the young mice were ready for testing, they showed detectable differences from normal young of their own strains. The important differences were in emotional responses. A tendency of the poor learners to 'freeze' in the shuttle-box was noticeably reduced by fostering, while the normally phlegmatic good learners were more emotional. But learning ability was scarcely affected by fostering. Hereditary good learners did very well in the shuttle-box, the poor learners poorly.

But now consider equally impressive evidence on the importance of environment. The performance of a young child at school is greatly influenced by what his teacher expects of him. We know that, from a somewhat underhand experiment, done in the mid-1960s by Robert Rosenthal of Harvard University and Lenore Jacobsen, herself a schoolteacher.

Rosenthal had found earlier that, if he told students that particular laboratory rats were either very bright or very stupid, the performance of the rats in maze-learning tests run by the students confirmed the prediction. The truth was that the rats were really all of the same strain. Evidently, the students treated the rats differently, in accordance with their expectations for them. The same proved to be the case for teachers and children.

The children at a San Francisco school were given a fanciful 'test of inflected acquisition' which was said to predict rapid development in some of the children. The teachers were later told, very casually, results of this 'test'. In fact the names of some of the children had been simply picked out at random.

Yet the prediction that these children would be 'spurters' turned out to be a self-fulfilling prophecy. Among the youngest children, the average gains in IQ scores in the ensuing academic year were twice as great for the named children as for their classmates. The teacher's expectation was signalled to the children, perhaps unwittingly, and the children became more confident in their own ability.

The problems confronting the serious inquirer into nature and nurture are well illustrated by the title of a recent learned paper: 'Are genetic correlations and environmental correlations correlated?' Perhaps the only way to make any sense of the conflicting information is to view the problem as Donald Hebb does. His answer to the nature-nurture riddle is '100 per cent heredity and 100 per cent environment'. If that seems cryptic, consider that a man has a height and a waist measurement, but that adding them together is meaningless. It may be equally meaningless to think of environmental effects as additions and subtractions on top of the gift of heredity. The genius of the genes and its evocation by the environment are both indispensable. In any case, haggling about IQ scores is a polemical luxury at a time when much of the potential of the human gene pool is being wasted for want of food.

The hungry brain

In large areas of Asia, Africa and Latin America, diets are unsatisfactory by normal medical standards, especially for lack of animal protein. Improvement in the past twenty years has been slight. Encouraging technical advances have included the growing of greatly improved cereals in tropical countries, but rapidly-increasing numbers of people tend to swallow the additional food produced, without improving the average diet. Uneven sharing of food means that, where statistical averages are poor, some plates are very empty indeed. Several million infants each year are taken seriously ill with diseases of malnutrition, such as kwashiorkor and marasmus. But more than half of all pre-school children in the developing countries, totalling an estimated 400 million, suffer milder but continuing malnutrition, as well as other diseases to which their weakened condition leaves them vulnerable. A visible stunting of body growth is one sign of this malnutrition, but the effects on the brain are harder to measure.

Researchers have to take human beings as they are, and cannot do controlled experiments. That means it is difficult to separate the effects of malnutrition from other factors. If a child in an impoverished village shows poor mental perfor-

238

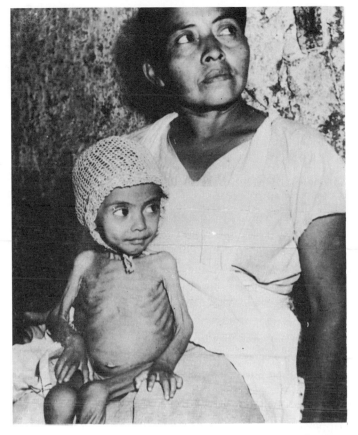

A young victim of malnutrition in Guatemala, where present studies are detecting lasting effects on mental capacity of inadequate feeding during infancy.

mance, it may be because he is badly fed. But it can also be a matter of heredity – he may come of a long line of dullards. Or perhaps he is brought up in unstimulating circumstances, like the American institutional children studied by White and Held. Elaborate field studies, like a series now in progress in Guatemala, have to be undertaken to find the facts. Joaquin Cravioto of Mexico City is one of the leaders of such work.

Meanwhile, looking into the effects of different diets on the brains and performance of animals gives quicker and more clear-cut results, but problems remain of how to interpret them. The brains of different animals mature at different times, in relation to day of birth. Anything discovered in a new-born rat, for example, would correspond to effects in humans before birth, because the rat's brain develops relatively late. In any case, the human brain is much more complex and subtle than the brains of experimental animals; consequences of brain damage by malnutrition may be either more serious or less serious in humans than in animals.

All these words of caution are necessary because of the gravity of the medical problem and its bearing on politics and economics. These are not only matters of curiosity or scientific

239

interest. Apart from their possible effects on policies for economic development, findings in this area may unintentionally give fresh ammunition for the racists to say, for example, 'Perhaps blacks don't have to be stupid, but they are because they've been badly fed'. With issues like this lurking in the background, we must be very careful in interpreting the results of the human tests and the animal experiments.

A variety of studies in children, in Yugoslavia, South Africa, India, Chile, Guatemala, Mexico and elsewhere, suggest that there is indeed a general effect of malnutrition on brain development. If the effect is real, it varies according to the age at which a child suffers the most severe lack of nourishment. Taking the results at their face value, deprivation below the age of 18 months does cause a permanent intellectual deficiency, implying that the fabric of the roof of the brain is damaged for life. Deprivation after 18 months has a different kind of effect. Mental capability is normal, but performance is poor, because the child is listless and inattentive; this effect is temporary and disappears if the child is properly fed.

The investigators take care, in their tests of perception and reasoning, to compare the malnourished children with other children of very similar family circumstances. All the complicating social factors mentioned before might leave more grounds for doubt about the importance of food, if there were not the supporting evidence of animal experiments. These reveal defects in the size, structure and chemistry of the brains of young animals raised on a low-protein diet, as well as showing that the animals perform relatively poorly at tasks such as maze-running.

By gross reckoning the brain does not suffer as badly as the rest of the body, at times of great hunger. It is as if nature has ordained that the all-important brain shall be spared as long as possible. For example, a three-month baby, dead of starvation, may have a body weight half the normal, yet his brain may be only about 15 per cent underweight. But this 'sparing' may not be completely successful, least of all at the periods when the brain is growing most rapidly. Dobbing and Sands, as mentioned earlier, have found that a peak in growth-rate of the human brain, when most of the neurons are formed, occurs in the period 15 to 20 weeks after conception – in other words, several months before birth.

That forces our attention to how malnutrition in the mother affects the baby. The mother supplies nourishment to the unborn child and removes waste products through the placenta and, in humans, malnutrition produces detectable changes in that organ. But, once again, animal experiments give more

240

explicit information. For example, working at the University of California, Los Angeles, Stephan Zamenhof and Edith van Marthens showed in the late 1960s that when female rats are kept on low-protein diets before mating and during pregnancy, the brains of the offspring were 25 per cent underweight. They were also deficient in the genetic material DNA to the extent of about 10 per cent – suggesting that one tenth of the neurons were simply missing.

The experimenters put the mothers back on an ordinary diet and allowed some of the young rats (first generation) to grow up fully nourished. The females were then mated with normal rats and went through pregnancy still well fed, to the delivery of their litters. These second-generation rats also turned out to be short of brain cells. But that may be merely an effect of reduced body size. Tests of maze-running performance now in progress at UCLA should show whether or not there is any effect on performance, due to malnutrition in the grandmother.

Putting the most modest interpretation on present evidence, there is a prima facie case for fearing a very harmful effect of inadequate feeding in the mother, or her baby, on the life-long mental powers of the child. A bolder interpretation is that a devastating assault on the minds of many millions of helpless individuals is occurring around the world. Making sure that pregnant women and babies were properly fed could probably save a great aggregate of human talent now being lost in the urine in the form of unreplaced nitrogen. Passing over the blight on individual lives, and looking only at communal needs, we may see a tragic inconsistency in striving to end illiteracy in regions where malnutrition occurs, without also taking steps to defend the young brains for which the education is intended.

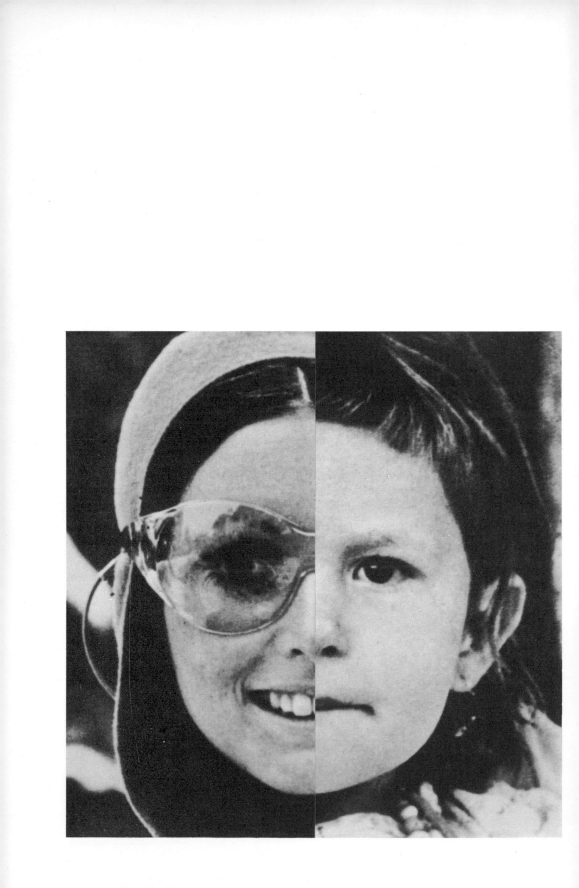

13 Left Mind, Right Mind

Separating the two big hemispheres at the top of the brain by surgery seemed to have no effect, until recent tests showed it produced two distinct minds under the one skull, with different qualities. This discovery renews the question of how the conscious mind is related to physical activities of the brain.

A housewife in her mid-thirties sits in a laboratory at the California Institute of Technology. In front of her is a screen and she has been asked to gaze at a spot marked in the middle of it. A strange picture appears briefly on the screen. It is a split face made up of two halves joined down the middle. On the right, as seen by the housewife, it is a young child; on the left a young woman wearing spectacles.

Next, the housewife is shown a choice of several faces, and she is asked to point with her right hand at the one she saw. She points at the picture of the young woman. She is then shown another composite face – a woman and an old man – and asked to say what she saw. She describes the old man and denies that there was anything odd about the picture.

Like the face on the screen, the housewife's brain has been split down the middle. She underwent an operation for

A split face (left), used in tests of patients whose brains have been surgically divided, is made up from two of the faces in the selection shown (right). The left side of the brain recognises the child, the right side, the woman in spectacles.

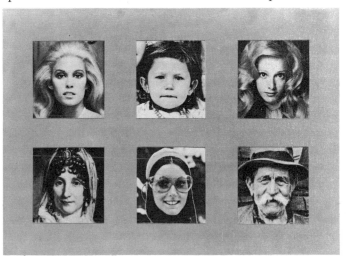

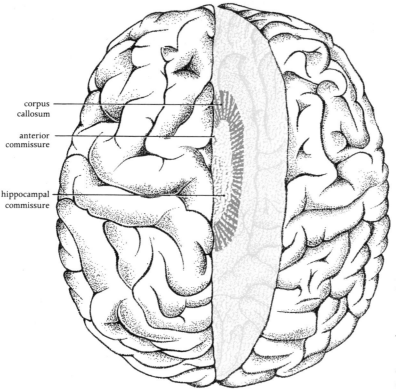

corpus
callosum

anterior
commissure

hippocampal
commissure

*Separating the hemispheres.
This view from above, with the
hemispheres pulled somewhat
apart, shows the cables of nerve
fibres which are cut in the split-
brain operation. (After
Gazzaniga). Below: after such an
operation, the housewife shows no
obvious disturbance of behaviour.*

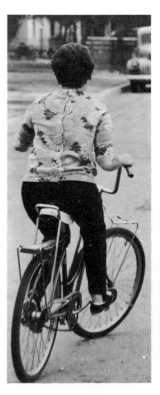

severe epilepsy in which the surgeon cut the great bundle of
nerve fibres which normally connect the two sides of the roof
of the brain. The operation was successful and the woman is
now able to lead a more normal life. To see her doing her house-
work, swimming, riding a bicycle, and so on, you would not
for one moment suppose there was anything unusual about
her. But the tests devised by Roger Sperry and his colleagues
show that she possesses two independent minds under the
one skull.

Of all the remarkable experiments and discoveries we encountered in our world-wide search for new knowledge about
the mind of man, the human split brain remains the most
haunting. It has, of course, nothing whatever to do with the
so-called 'split personality' of some mental patients. The split-
brain patient possesses a truly split mind. The demonstration
that zones of perception, decision-making and consciousness
have been divided by the surgeon provides the most forcible
evidence of the unity of brain and mind that medical science is
ever likely to give to the doubting onlooker.

In the test with the faces, just described, the housewife saw
the woman with the right side of her brain and the old man with
244   the left side. That is because of the way the nerve fibres from

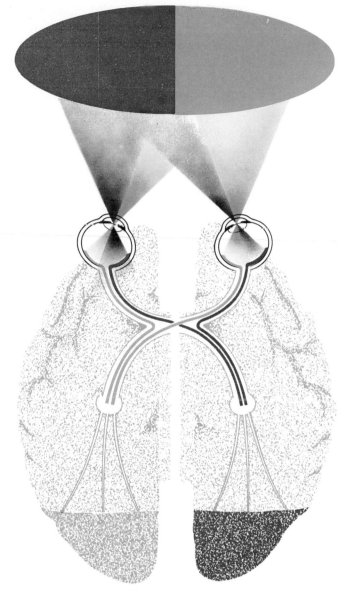

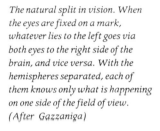

The natural split in vision. When the eyes are fixed on a mark, whatever lies to the left goes via both eyes to the right side of the brain, and vice versa. With the hemispheres separated, each of them knows only what is happening on one side of the field of view. (After Gazzaniga)

the corresponding regions of both eyes are divided between the two hemispheres of the brain (see the diagram above). With her gaze fixed upon the marked spot, and the picture appearing fleetingly, there was no sharing of information by movement of the eyes. The split in the brain prevented the normal interchange of information between the two sides of the brain.

Each side of the brain was thus blind to what the other side was seeing. The left side of the brain controls speech so, when the housewife was asked to tell what she had seen, she naturally reported the old man and his hat. The explanation of

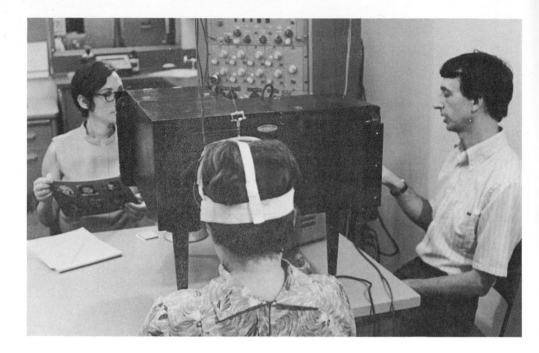

why, in the first test, she pointed with her right hand at the picture of the woman is more subtle. It is normal to think that the right hand is controlled by the left side of the brain, as a result of the grand cross-over of functions; therefore you might expect it to point out the child. But the right side of the brain can also guide the eyes and either hand, for pointing purposes, and it turns out to be better at recognising faces than the left side of the brain is; so it had its way, and selected the picture of the young woman in spectacles which it had seen on the screen.

The test with the faces was a new one, when the housewife underwent it in 1970, but she had been co-operating with Sperry for several years previously. She is one of a small number of such patients, mostly former epileptics, who have helped Caltech investigators find out what is abnormal about them. By outward appearances, nothing is wrong. When brain surgeons began carrying out split-brain operations in the late 1930s, they reported that there was no detectable effect after the operation, except relief of the epilepsy for which it was done. In other words, the mass of fibres connecting the two sides of the roof of the brain served no discernible purpose except to help epileptic seizures spread across the brain.

The break came in 1951, when a young colleague of Sperry, Ronald Myers, showed that an animal with a split brain and with vision also split could learn opposite solutions to the

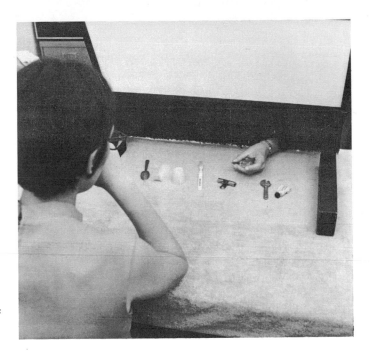

The housewife (back to camera, left) looks into the apparatus where the split faces are projected. Her headgear checks against head movements. Right : the housewife's left hand feels for objects that she cannot see

same experimental test, using the two halves of his brain. Since then, Sperry and his group have explored the worlds of the split brain in animals, and more recently in man.

The music of the hemispheres

When our Californian housewife is asked to use her left hand to feel objects behind a screen, and to name them, she cannot do so. Her right brain is mute. But the right-brain/left-hand combination is more skilled than its partner in recognising objects by feeling them, provided it can identify them otherwise than by words. The two brains of the split-brain patient are thus very different in character. It follows that each of us has similarly contrasting brains within his own head, although the effects are almost completely masked by the normal co-operation of the two sides of the brain.

From worms to humans, one of the recurring themes in the design of animals is symmetry of left and right. Saw us down the middle and prop one half against the mirror, and we shall seem whole again. We have two eyes, two lungs, two kidneys and so on, and though we have only one mouth, it precisely straddles the midline. Some organs, including the heart and the gut, are asymmetrical in their connections but these irregularities are not visible from the outside.

An exposed brain is symmetrical to the casual eye. Indeed its symmetry is emphasised by the prominent fore-and-aft fissure in the roof separating the two hemispheres of the cerebral cortex like a line of meridian. Symmetry is preserved in the cross-overs in information flowing in and out of the brain, with the left hemisphere having main responsibility for the right side of the body, and vice versa. In the normal brain, the fibres of the so-called 'hard body' (corpus callosum), and other deep-lying connection points, ensure abundant interchange of information, so that the left hand knows what the right hand doeth.

In the last few years even the superficial symmetry of the human brain has been falsified by measurements mentioned earlier (p. 140). Regions involved in speech, on the left side of the brain, are bigger than corresponding regions on the right. The functional differences have been known for much longer, of course, not only in the special role of the left brain in language but also in the common ascendancy of the left-brain/right-hand combination in handwriting and in other skilled tasks.

A digression about left-handers (and I write as one myself): precious little is known for certain about why one person in 14 or thereabouts is perverse in this respect or, for that matter, why 13 out of 14 are right-handed. In rats and some other animals, there is a dominant hand, but it is equally likely to be right or left. The fact that right-handedness is the norm in humans is probably connected with the occurrence of the speech area in the left of the brain. Some natural left-handers have their speech areas on the 'wrong' side of the brain but, according to Wilder Penfield, most left-handers are normal in that respect. It is not even clear whether left-handedness is hereditary, or is due to a defect in the left brain or some other unflattering physical or psychological cause.

After the apparently drastic operation of cutting the connections between the two hemispheres, patients were able unconsciously to fool the eminent experts because they lacked any obvious disability. In ordinary everyday situations, there is plenty of opportunity for the two hemispheres to discover independently what is going on. Naturally, they then co-operate. The eyes are very important when, for example, the split-brain housewife is cooking. In any case, a little information does pass to and fro between the left hemisphere of the brain and the left side of the body, and similarly on the right. Only in carefully contrived tests is detailed information confined to one hemisphere or the other.

Otherwise, any disability seems to be less unpleasant or inconvenient than the severe epilepsy which prompted the operation. There are rare cases in which individuals are born lacking the main connecting fibres between the hemispheres. Sperry once had occasion to test such a person, a girl student, and found no detectable consequence of this congenital defect. Evidently, in childhood, while the brain was still immature, it reorganised its operations to compensate for its peculiarity – an interesting sidelight on that argument about nature and nurture!

Two surgeons working at the California College of Medicine began to employ the split-brain treatment in humans, from 1961 onwards. Sperry, with Michael Gazzaniga and other colleagues, then had convenient opportunities to study the effects. In the period following the operation the whole of the left of the patient's body seemed to be very inactive and insensitive, but gradually the right side of the brain began to awaken to its unaccustomed independence. Thereafter it was possible to test, besides the effects of disconnection, the inherent powers of the two hemispheres. As we all possess the same double brain structure, it is no disrespect to the unlucky patients who supply this knowledge, if we give nicknames to the two hemispheres.

Dexter and Lefty

So let me introduce Dexter and Lefty, two brothers as unlike as Jacob and Esau. Dexter, dwelling in the left of the head but controlling the right hand, is the smart one who does all the talking. Conversing with a split-brain patient, it's Dexter that you meet; Lefty stands by quietly, listening politely to what is said but saying nothing. Nor does he do anything much, unless directly asked to carry out a task. No one can say what induced Lefty to give up his birthright of command of language, because all the evidence suggests that, at the age of three, his competence was equal to his brother's.

Dexter can read and write fluently and does the difficult arithmetic. Lefty, though dumb, is not entirely illiterate. He can read common words, do simple arithmetic, and understand most of what is said to him. For example, with the left hand groping among objects in a bag out of sight, a split-brain patient can respond to the instruction, 'Retrieve the fruit monkeys like best,' by pulling out a plastic banana. And in many tests, the patient is asked to say what the left hand is feeling; Dexter simply has no idea and makes a guess, where-

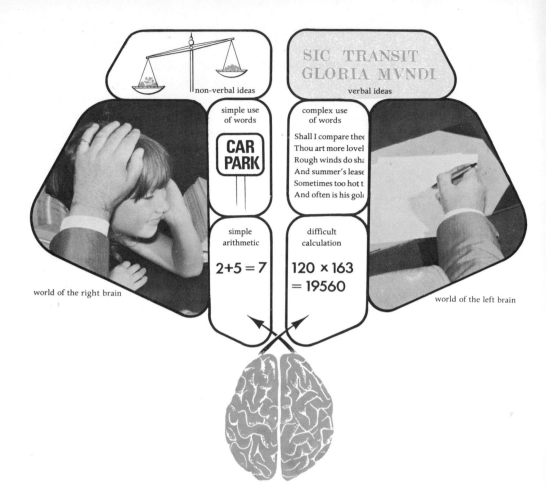

non-verbal ideas

simple use
of words

CAR
PARK

simple
arithmetic

$2+5=7$

SIC TRANSIT
GLORIA MVNDI
verbal ideas

complex use
of words

Shall I compare thee
Thou art more lovel
Rough winds do sha
And summer's lease
Sometimes too hot t
And often is his gol

difficult
calculation

120×163
$= 19560$

world of the right brain

world of the left brain

The worlds of the left and right hemispheres of the brain. These differences occur, although concealed, in normal brains.

upon Lefty frowns and shakes their common head. 'Oh no, I'm wrong,' says Dexter.

Lefty certainly seems less bright than Dexter, in the adult, but he is far from stupid. In tests of perception, comprehension and memory, where he can make non-verbal responses, he performs very well. In double tasks of a simple kind, such as searching for different objects or reacting to different signals with the two hands, Lefty and Dexter go their ways independently and the patient can complete the task more rapidly than a normal person could. But Sperry is careful to deny that patients are actually better off with their split brains!

And Lefty has the keener sense of shape, form and texture. He can, for example, copy a geometrical picture much more accurately than Dexter can – the lines are clumsier but essential features are not omitted as they are liable to be when Dexter tries his hand. Faced with evidence of Lefty's deeds Dexter may say, 'Well, I must have done it unconsciously'.

Perhaps Lefty's education has been grievously neglected. Here is fully half of the human cerebral cortex which is relegated to the status of a second-class citizen. He may represent a great waste of mental capacity, left poorly nurtured. As Sperry nowadays urges upon anyone willing to listen, the educational systems of many nations are immensely biased in their reliance on verbal inputs and outputs. We should be paying much more attention than we do to the cultivation of non-verbal skills at school.

In a series of tests of the split-brain patients done in co-operation with the Montreal Neurological Institute, basic mechanisms underlying normal hearing were in question. Unlike the eyes (each of which feeds half its information to one side of the brain and half to the other), both ears send all their information to both sides. But as the tests in the split-brain patients confirmed, each side of the brain listens more intently to the ear on the opposite side of the head, and suppresses information from its near ear if there is any conflict. In a test of verbal responses (by Dexter) different sets of numbers were presented to the two ears simultaneously through headphones; most of the split-brain patients reported hearing nothing at all in the left ear. In a test calling for action by the left hand (by Lefty), instructions given in the left ear were obeyed but other instructions given simultaneously in the right ear were often neglected.

Even in the Californian patients the brain is not completely split. Although the severing of connections between the two

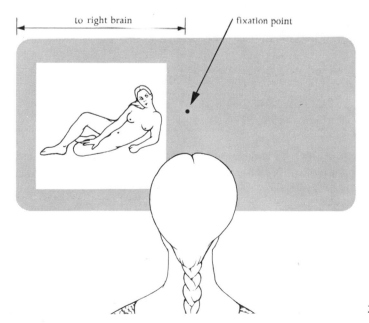

Shared emotions. The left side of the brain is unable to explain the feelings produced by the picture of the nude, which it has not seen.

to right brain   fixation point

sides of the upper brain has been particularly thorough, the hemispheres are united via the brain stem. Factual information does not seem to flow by that route, but emotional effects can do so. This produces one of the strangest reactions of all. The patient is staring at the mark on the screen and pictures of geometrical figures are being flashed on the screen. Unexpectedly, a nude pin-up appears on the left, for the attention of the right hemisphere. The talkative left brain testifies that nothing has been seen, but the patient begins to chuckle. Asked why, the left brain replies, 'I don't know – oh, that funny machine'.

Some seek to avoid the disturbing implications of the split in consciousness in the split-brain patient, by describing the mute side as a mindless automaton – thereby ascribing consciousness only to one side of the brain. But to find out what goes on in the mute hemisphere, and what is the quality of its mental life, has been an important objective in the Caltech

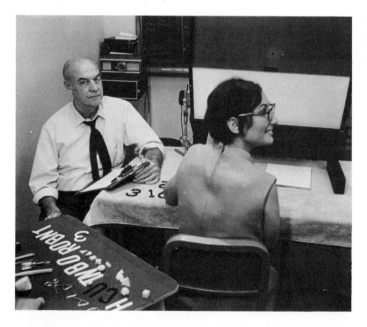

Roger Sperry: 'Surgical division of the brain also divides the mind into two separate realms of human consciousness.'

tests. Sperry himself is satisfied that an independent stream of consciousness, characteristically human, is operating there and that consciousness resides in the tissue of both cerebral hemispheres.

Mind as spirit

'I think, therefore I am.' René Descartes' declaration of more than three centuries ago asserted self-consciousness as evidence of the existence of God and the immortality of the soul.

To attempt to run through what the sages of Western philosophy from Plato onwards have had to say about the relationships of God, soul, mind, brain and body would take us too far from the present-day argument. To provide some perspective for current issues it may be sufficient to pick out some contrasting points of view which are taken seriously today, beginning with Descartes, the most influential philosopher since Aristotle and the man from whom the modern interest in the mind-brain problem most plainly flows. Though his detailed arguments seem quaint, no one has since succeeded in entirely ridding us of the idea that the mind and brain are quite distinct.

Descartes regarded living things as automatic machines – thus far, he was very modern. But animals did not talk, so evidently they had no souls. From that, it followed that the soul was something extra, independent of the animal-like human body. Body and mind operated in different worlds, so separate that thoughts could not affect anything in the physical world.

Descartes compromised a little on this matter of will, although those who followed him quickly corrected his inconsistency. Moreover, Descartes, who was really very mechanically minded, visualised the soul sitting in the middle of the head, at the pineal gland. Despite these lapses, the general sense of Descartes' argument was unmistakable: mind was mind and brain was brain, and never the twain should meet. Even people whose views on the soul are quite opposed to Descartes' have drawn sustenance from him, because his dichotomy allows them to exclude all consideration of the mind from their 'real' world.

Continuing belief in the divine origins of the human mind is certainly not incompatible with the findings of brain research up to this time – the uncertainties are still ample to accommodate that possibility. Sir John Eccles is one leading researcher who has been at pains to make his convictions clear:

> I believe that there is a fundamental mystery in my personal existence, transcending the biological account of the development of my body and my brain. That belief, of course, is in keeping with the religious concept of the soul and with its special creation by God.

In our time Gilbert Ryle of Oxford has mocked Descartes' view of the mind as 'the ghost in the machine'. In Ryle's opinion, all the worry about the status of the mind arises because people assign mental life to the wrong logical category. Saying that mental processes occur does not mean the same sort of thing as saying that physical processes occur. Ryle offers the parable of a foreigner visiting Oxford who asks, after a tour of the colleges, libraries, laboratories and so on, 'But where is the University?' The 'University' (at least in a dispersed institution like Oxford) is not in the same category as the colleges; similarly 'mind' is not in the same category as 'body'.

Intelligent performance, Ryle says, is not a clue to the workings of the mind; it *is* the workings of the mind. Thinking, feeling and willing are not isolated parts of the mind: emotion is a combination of feeling and willing while the will works in harness with reasoning and feeling. Consciousness is not a privileged access into the workings of one's mind. Psychologists will do well if they can scotch the idea of a special mind-stuff, although Ryle does not favour the view that a man is just a higher mammal. 'There has yet to be ventured the hazardous leap to the hypothesis that perhaps he is a man.'

When he published this analysis in 1949, Ryle expected to be misunderstood and to have his plea of logic disallowed as mere subterfuge. Certainly he seemed to be trying to dispose of a real problem by a verbal trick, although his contention was that the problem was only verbal to start with. In any case, in practical effect, Ryle's arguments have not visibly dislodged the mentalists and materialists from their established positions. These are the thinkers, so prominent in the first half of this century, who have evaded the mind-brain issue either by considering mental processes without reference to the brain or by denying the importance, or even the existence, of the conscious mind. Their positions are well illustrated by two conspicuous schools of psychology – the one derived from Sigmund Freud of Vienna, the other from Ivan Pavlov of St Petersburg.

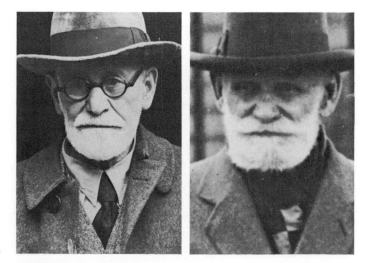

Sigmund Freud (left): 'We have decided to assume the existence of only two basic instincts, Eros and the destructive instinct.'

For I. P. Pavlov (right), behaviour was a matter of conditioned responses.

Freud was a physician, a neurologist by training, who found himself treating the psychologically sick. As a former laboratory scientist, he looked for precise explanations of mental disorders, much as a pathologist seeks the microbe or the block that causes physical disease. But, confronted with suffering individuals and listening to their words rather than their heart beats, Freud could not postpone action until academic research had caught up with the problems of mental function. He jumped in at the deep end of the psychic pool. He found it deeper than anyone had supposed, with a great zone of unconscious mental life influencing our conduct.

Thereafter, Freud constructed the psychoanalytical theory of mental processes, completely divorced from any specifiable brain mechanisms, although it drew on the metaphor of a machine. The unconscious, or id, was the power source of the human personality, where instincts, especially of sex and aggression, created energy (libido) and unpleasant emotional tension. The mind as a whole operated for the relief of tension, and success was accompanied by conscious pleasure. Provided the conscious mind, or ego, assisted the id towards gratification, it could draw upon the limited supply of instinctual energy. But this id-ego engine was governed by the superego, embodying ideals and conscience, whereby the demands of society were built into the mind of the individual citizen. The mind also had a variety of defence mechanisms for reducing anxiety.

With some notable exceptions, most followers of Freud have not attempted to relate this model of mental action, or its subsequent elaborations, to the physical workings of the brain. No

The Freudian world is full of symbolism. The jar, for example, is a female symbol, and so are the wagons, while the locomotive is 'male'. The way a boy plays with a train is held to show his attitude to his parents and his own masculinity.

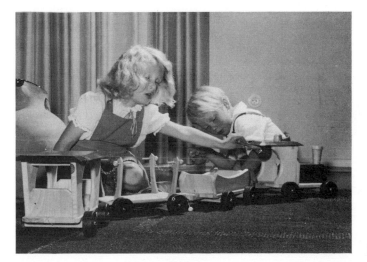

one has proposed, for example, looking for the flow of instinctual energy with micro-electrodes. Their mental engine is an abstract one, like a theory in economics. And, although well-informed psychoanalysts are naturally interested in the discoveries of the brain researchers, they see them in contrast with their own role, as it is expressed by Tom Main of London:

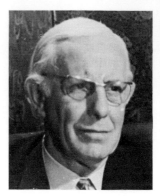

> I deal in concepts such as envy and triumph, grief and joy, revenge and remorse. These matters of mind are no less real than molecules or brain cells. Indeed, in terms of man's daily experience and troubles, they are more important and they need study. Today's emphasis on atomic sciences and methods, and their mimicry by biologists, poses a needless threat to our humanity if it leads men away from their own inner awareness just because it can't be put under some microscope.

Tom Main, psychoanalyst :
'Matters of mind are no less real
than molecules or brain cells.'

Psychologists experimenting with animals in the tradition of Pavlov were remarkably adept at using their minds to deny the existence of their minds. In complete contrast with the Freudians, they declared themselves to be concerned only with the outward manifestations of cerebral operations – the response evoked by a stimulus. As an experimental tactic it was deservedly successful; by refusing to assume any more complex an inner process than was necessary to explain the experimental observations, this approach was scientifically more convincing than the vague, untestable propositions of introspective psychology. Untold legions of dogs, rats and pigeons salivated, pressed levers and pecked in comforting conformity with predictions from very simple principles, thereby proving, allegedly, that all behaviour was a mixture of conditioned reflexes.

Pavlov discovered the conditioned reflex during his great researches on digestion in dogs. He himself was quite prepared to speculate about inner processes of excitation and inhibition going on unobserved in the brains of his dogs, although only in materialistic terms. Consciousness was out; and in the United States, too, John B. Watson and his successors found in the conditioned reflex the way of taking the psyche out of psychology in calling it behaviourism. When trial-and-error learning with reinforcement greatly extended the scope of experimental conditioning, the behaviourists entered their heyday and B. F. Skinner was their prophet. In 1970, Skinner expressed his view thus:

> We do not need to create a duplicate of the brain, called
> the mind. We can deal with the brain in other ways . . . The

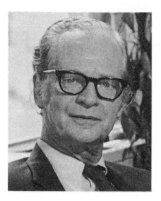

B. F. Skinner, behaviourist:
'We can deal with
the brain in other ways.'

behaviourist does not ignore consciousness, as is often said. He simply deals in other ways with the facts that are said to show that a person is conscious. In explaining these and other facts he emphasises what has happened to a person during his lifetime. Naturally the brain plays an important role in bridging the gap between what has happened to a person and his current behaviour. Eventually the physiologist will tell us how the brain does this but we cannot wait for him, because we must get on with the analysis and in particular with applying it to the solution of problems in the world today.

But even as Skinner and his colleagues were rising to a peak of influence in the United States, the situation was changing. Psychobiology and neuropsychology – under these and other names, new bridges were being built between the knowledge of psychology and the knowledge of brain systems. Since about 1950, their footing in biology growing firmer, some leading experimental psychologists have confidently declared the stimulus-response formula inadequate for explaining conduct. Even as 'private' a phenomenon as dreaming became amenable to laboratory observation while, on the other hand, attempts to mimic human mental powers with computers met salutary difficulties. The oversimplified views of the past have been a product of scientific specialisation; with more pooling of knowledge, the richness and grandeur of the brain and its accomplishments have become plainer.

Specialisation has hazards other than simple ignorance. The tendency to lump certain opinions together is a vice that philosophers and scientists share with politicians; indeed, it tells us something about the way the human mind works. Men who believe, as rationalist followers of Descartes, that the royal road to knowledge is by deductive reasoning, are also inclined to assign to the conscious mind a special status in nature and to believe that mental powers are inborn.

Their rivals are empiricists, who rely upon learning about nature by experiment and inductive reasoning. They are more liable to see themselves and their fellow men as overgrown rats trying to master mazes by trial and error and to suppose that consciousness is unimportant; it also comes more easily to them to picture the mind of a child as a clean slate, to be filled by experience as learned journals are filled by experimental results.

In short, the method biases the conclusion. That is human enough but the result is a confusion of issues as unforgivable as that of the politician who deals in the same breath with student demonstrators, illegal immigrants and women seeking abortions. Disentangling the issues is not too difficult, and it may encourage a more open mind to what the answers may be. The first two questions are peripheral to the problem of consciousness, the second two are central:

1. Which is the better strategy for enlarging human knowledge – reasoning from pre-existing knowledge, or careful observation and experiment?
2. To what extent is human ability inherited, to what extent is it acquired? (Here are the issues of innateness of language and of nature versus nurture, discussed in the previous chapters.)
3. What is the status of consciousness: an unimportant 'epiphenomenon', a functionally important cerebral mechanism, or the only important reality?
4. What is the relationship between consciousness and brain mechanisms: indistinguishable, closely linked, loosely linked, separate but coexistent, or separate (with consciousness able to exist outside the body, e.g. after death)?

There is, of course, some coupling between some of the possible answers to these questions. It would not make much sense, for example, to say that consciousness is both unimportant and immortal. But the coupling is much weaker than the fortified positions adopted by the rival schools of thought would suggest, and weakest of all in the middle ground where the correct answers are most likely to lie.

Two kinds of explanation

Psychological researchers need to generate explanations of what they find, to hold their ideas together. Jean Piaget of Geneva has checked off, in systematic fashion, the ways that are open to them. His selection of the two most useful forms of explanation helps to define the problem of relating conscious experience to physical processes in the brain.

One form is the 'organic reductionism', which attempts to find the processes at work in the brain; for some lower forms of conduct it may provide a very complete explanation. But for the higher forms of conduct, including those involving self-awareness, it is necessary to go in for 'construction' – essentially the making of abstract theories which propose psychological laws and schemes of cause and effect. The construction is not, in the first instance, based on the details of any particular brain system.

These approaches need not conflict; rather, the problem is to unite them, to relate a conscious idea to the brain system which makes the idea possible. The big question is whether or not the link between them is 'causal' or not – whether there is interaction between the brain and consciousness, or whether they are simply parallel but different phenomena unable to affect one another.

Piaget himself denies the possibility of interaction. Consciousness, being intangible and without force, cannot act upon the brain in any way. But he also rejects other opinions, that the mind has a quite separate existence of its own, or that consciousness is just an awareness of certain activities in the brain. Piaget is convinced by his studies of the development of conscious thought in children and in human history that consciousness must have a function. The solution to the riddle that he offers is a role for consciousness in recognising, in a wholly abstract sense, the truth or falsehood of propositions generated by the operations of the brain, and their implications. In the long run, to reconcile consciousness and brain, Piaget expects the explanations of 'organic reductionism' and the theoretical models of 'construction' to turn out to be essentially the same.

Consciousness is thus left, by Piaget, as a kind of ethereal, mathematically-minded critic of physical events in the brain. It may be too close to the old idea of a semi-detached soul for modern taste. My mental critic is not persuaded by Piaget of the truth of its own existence, at least in the abstract form he suggests. Can his two kinds of psychological explanation, 'reductionist' and 'constructive', be linked in any more down-to-earth way?

In this connection, I shall summarise two more opinions about the relationship of consciousness to the rest of the brain's operations. Both of them emerged in the late 1960s. Roger Sperry and Ulric Neisser have been mentioned frequently enough in this book to need no further testimonials, as people in the thick of current experiment and theory, while it is Sperry's split-brain work that has prompted this digression into philosophy.

They are both level-headed men who have not been intimidated by the mid-century orthodoxy which made consciousness almost a taboo subject for experimental psychologists. Both acknowledge a debt to the Gestalt psychologists of the inter-war years. My motive in giving preference to their views is simply that of a reporter who sees in them serious attempts to reach the same objective as his own: that of beginning to account for the human mind of personal experience, in the light of current discoveries about brain mechanisms.

Although Piaget says it is impossible, Sperry proposes a practical reaction of consciousness upon the physical workings of the brain. Conscious thoughts are not merely passive, impotent echoes of the firing patterns of the brain circuits. Nor are they, as the orthodoxy would have it, without any bearing on human performance and conduct. Sperry puts consciousness to work and gives it 'a reason for having evolved'. The two distinct zones of consciousness which he is satisfied he finds in the split-brain patients persuade him that consciousness is inseparable from brain tissue. But it is something more than the sum of the physical events of the brain.

By its consciousness, the brain monitors its own activities – not scrutinising the actions of individual cells, but detecting overall qualities of different activity patterns. The conscious properties of the brain, Sperry says, 'encompass and transcend the details of nerve impulse traffic in the cerebral networks in the same way that the properties of the organism transcend the properties of its cells'. And consciousness influences the working of the brain. Sperry is careful to say that it does not 'intervene' to alter the laws for the generation or transmission of nerve impulses. Rather, it 'supervenes', by requiring that the brain's activity operates within an envelope of larger configurations, much as the drops of water swirl in an eddy in a stream.

'In the human head there are forces within forces within forces, as in no other cubic half-foot of the universe that we know.' Sperry does not offer to explain *how* consciousness is built from the mechanisms of the brain – finding this out becomes the central challenge for the future. But he suspects that the essential features of organisation that accomplish it are built into the brain and are switched on by the arousal system in the brain stem.

Sperry's opinion falls in the middle of the spectrum of older ideas about mind and brain. He assigns practical power to mental activity but denies that it can exist apart from the brain processes – in other words, there is no immortal soul, no extrasensory perception. The other viewpoint I would pick out is by no means incompatible with Sperry's. While Sperry tries to span the whole range of 'forces within forces' in the human head, Ulric Neisser is more concerned with the details of certain psychological processes. In particular he suggests how the highest processes can be built from essential and elementary activities, such as perceiving, acting and remembering.

Neisser allows for a distinct process of executive control of thinking, but denies that this need imply a 'little man' sitting inside the head. The information stored in the memory represents traces of previous activity, whether mental or overt. As a first step towards using it for recall or for thinking, the brain processes a flood of these traces into crudely-formed thoughts. But these are transient and ill-organised, very like the flood of information from the eyes before the brain has formed the idea of what it is seeing.

A second step is needed for the accomplishment of directed thought and deliberate recall. Again it is like a visual process, the focusing of the attention on the required idea. There is manipulation of the available information, much as the eye-brain system picks out features of special interest in the visual scene. Here is where the 'executive' comes in. The process is not altogether unlike the work of the consciousness as critic, as described by Piaget, but it is in closer control of events than Piaget allows.

Indeed, action by the 'executive' is necessary for the most rudimentary of mental operations, such as remembering. Some mechanism has to pick out wanted information from the memory, a mechanism which is different from the memory itself. But it does not have to be a 'little man'. No one suggests that there is a 'little man' inside a computer, yet it is quite normal to operate a computer in a comparable way, with an executive program which intervenes to decide which of the other available programs should be used in given circumstances.

Although the comparison helps Neisser out of a philosophical impasse, he does not think the brain is much like a computer. The program of the brain's executive is not written by a programmer. Like many other processes in the brain, it is learnt by experience. The course of its constructive operations is governed by motives and expectations as well as by the contents of the memory. We cannot attempt to predict what a person will think of next, unless we know what he is trying to do and why. 'For this reason,' Neisser concludes, 'a really satisfactory theory of the higher mental processes can only come into being when we also have theories of motivation, personality, and social interaction.'

In ideas such as these, a compromise offers itself as the solution to the Cartesian dilemma. We need neither glorify the conscious mind as the immortal soul, nor denigrate it as unimportant because it is not readily susceptible to objective investigation. Instead we simply stop being coy about it and take the conscious mind as a matter of fact.

Various elements of our conscious experience arise, as we have seen, out of active systems essential to the rudimentary functions of the brain: waking and attending, perceiving and remembering, acting and deciding, planning and imagining. *Why* these operations should feel, subjectively, the way they do may be a question of ultimate cause as refractory as asking why the universe exists. But that is no excuse for doubting the reality of consciousness, as a characteristic of living brain tissue as rich as ours. It is a product of physical mechanism much as the capricious symmetry of a snowflake is an emergent quality of ice crystals which cannot be explained simply in terms of chemical forces in the water molecules. There is no reason, in theory, why an artificial machine of sufficient complexity should not also be conscious.

Waiting for Gödel

If a psychical theory of the twenty-second century should prove consciousness to be an inevitable consequence of certain laws of complex systems, you would still have to explain why those laws existed. The over-persistent seeker of ultimate causes may be, to paraphrase Bernard Shaw, the unsceptical in full pursuit of the unknowable.

At this instant of a primitive era, the trend in brain research is away from the grandiose, overarching theories of 1900 – 1950, towards a more liberal philosophy. It is not a retreat into the supernatural – far from it. The discovery of palpable mechanisms in the brain, which make good sense to man the engineer, encourages the conviction that mental powers are to be explained in terms of such mechanisms.

A declaration, in the spirit of this book, that the mind is the brain is a machine, may avert more dangerous kinds of simple-mindedness. It is a fantastic machine which integrates, in its circuits and its chemistry, two billion years of biological evolution, 50,000 years of cultural evolution and the lifetime of personal evolution of each one of us. To say that we are nothing but a set of conditioned reflexes and that our conscious thoughts are of no account is as absurd as to share the opposite view of those who would detach our mental experience from the brain and consider it without regard to conditioned reflexes and subtler mechanisms that mediate the experience.

Though no mystic, Noam Chomsky suspects that the mechanisms of mind are far beyond the reach of present-day physics and chemistry. That may be true, in the last resort. But science is not a textbook which must be complete before it can be printed. It is a process of discovery, a game played by successive generations of young men for its own sake and for the help it can give along the way to the community at large. Finding out matters more than knowing.

There are also grave mathematical reasons for suspecting that we can never fully comprehend our own minds. A famous theorem of Kurt Gödel says that a mathematical system cannot be completely self-descriptive; all the rules necessary for describing the system cannot be stated within the system. The human brain is a system presumably conforming with mathematical law; therefore, the argument goes, it can never contain a complete account of itself. Roger Sperry's retort, when people show signs of letting Gödel get them down, is to say: 'Underline that word *complete*, and then consider the explanatory possibilities that remain; also underline *itself* and remember that this logic does not prevent a man's mind from acquiring a complete description of his neighbour's mind.'

I would liken twentieth-century brain research to sixteenth-century astronomy. We are the privileged onlookers in a Copernican phase when men are putting their conscious experience into orbit around the brain. We may be waiting for the Isaac Newton of the nervous system who will reveal what holds this universe together but I doubt if events will work out quite like that. In any case, the cosmos as comprehended by Newton fell very far short, both in mechanism and in grandeur, of the universe as perceived with modern telescopes and illuminated by modern physics. So even if men of great insight astound us in the years ahead, their discoveries about the brain may leave much unexplained or unexplored.

Astronomers have now reached out to an edge beyond which the universe is unobservable in principle – their equivalent of Gödel – so that discovery in astronomy may peter out in the next century or two. The mind of man, though bounded by a nutshell, is king of a conceptual space more truly infinite than the material universe. Moreover, that space is different for every human individual. For that reason, there can be no end to the possibility of discovery in psychology, so long as mankind survives.

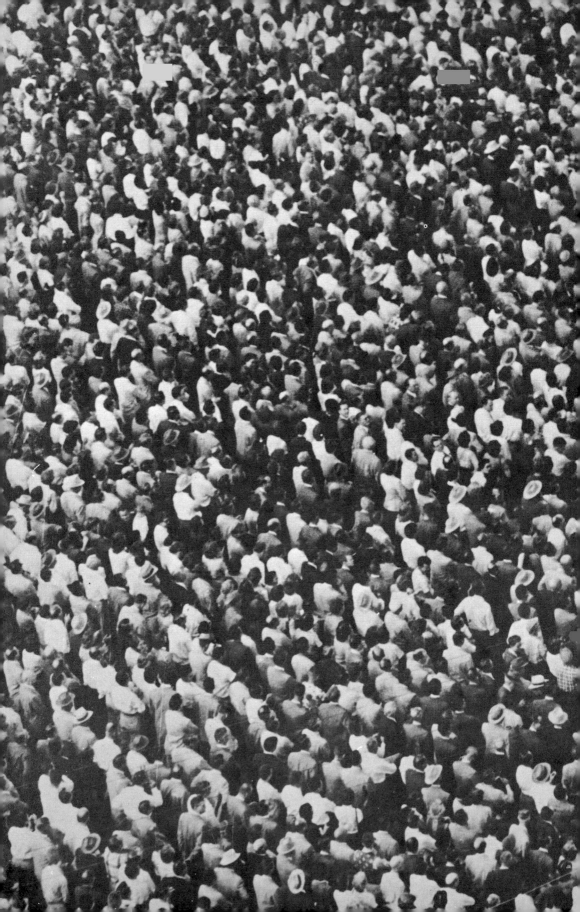

14   Is Man Obsolete?

The fashion is for self-denigration, and for suggestions for altering or superseding human nature; but such prescriptions overlook the subtle balance of reason and emotion built into our minds over long periods. Man has adapted to many changes – must he now learn to live without glib theories?

In a laboratory in Edinburgh, a robot contemplated a teacup. The machine turned the teacup round and drew it closer to its eye (a television camera) for a different view, acting much as a child would do when peeping at a strange object. This was one trial in an effort to teach the robot to recognise teacups. Other teacups, coming in various shapes, sizes and colours, were presented to the machine.

For Donald Michie and his colleagues, in Edinburgh University's department of machine intelligence and perception, the robot embodied and tested current ideas about how to

Thanks to our mental powers the human species has prospered and multiplied, but our numbers and our rate of consumption of the earth's resources have now become alarming.

Right: Members of the Edinburgh machine-intelligence team, with Donald Michie (centre). Cups and spectacles are among the objects that the robot is to recognise.

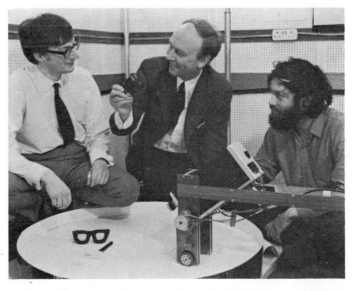

make a computer behave intelligently. With just a turntable and a camera, the robot fell far short of the popular idea of a robot, all thrashing arms and flashing lights. The essence of the   265

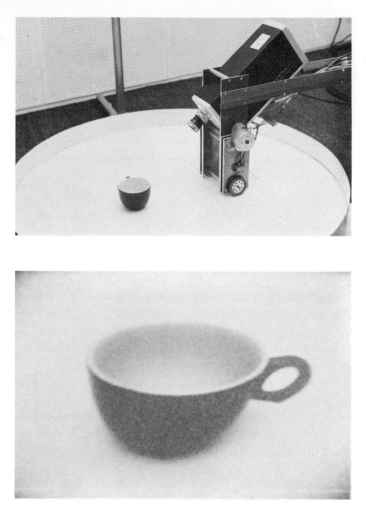

Successive stages in the analysis of a cup by the Edinburgh Mark I robot. Left: the robot's television camera observes the cup on the rotatable viewing platform. Centre: the robot's-eye view, as displayed on a monitor. Bottom left: first analysis of the pattern by the computer, with symbols for 16 different levels of brightness. The next step (bottom, right) is to analyse the object into different regions. The hole in the handle is marked with 'C's and the bottom shadow is distinguished from the cup proper. Then (opposite) the machine proceeds to compute relations between the regions, some of which are indicated here, including 'compactness' and 'adjacency'. Other objects, spectacles for example, will show quite different relations between regions.

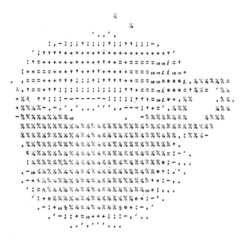

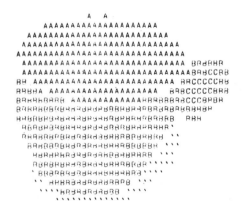

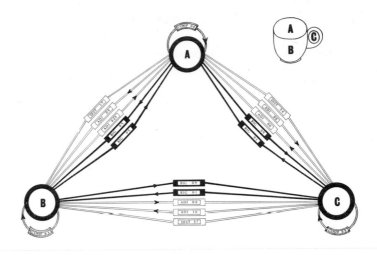

Edinburgh machine was in another room, a computer set to analyse information from the camera 'eye' and gradually to formulate the abstract concept of a teacup, regardless of the variations between teacups. Such ability, which seems so natural to human beings, is achieved in a computer only by ingenious programming.

When computers first appeared on the scene, in the 1940s, journalists named them 'electronic brains'. Then a reaction set in; nowadays the usual thing to say is that a computer is a moronic calculator. Despite their enormous speed of calculation and their ability to carry out logical operations at high speed, they depend completely on the people who write their programs, for all their clever tricks. A human slip can completely frustrate a computer. You may not be much perturbed by the fact that their are several mipsprints and other mistake in this sentence but equivalant errors in a computer program could reduce a mighty machine to impotence.

That is one reason why a small band of experimenters around the world are interested in artificial intelligence – in the attempt to make machines that think for themselves. These men have to try to define thought processes as practical mechanisms. They take it for granted, of course, that there is nothing supernatural about thought. They believe that a machine can, in theory, react in a manner indicating it is thinking and solving problems in much the same way that humans think. When pressed to define what he has in mind, the artificial-intelligence specialist may reply that he wants a machine that can do well in an IQ test.

If you say of someone that 'he jumps to conclusions' you probably mean it abusively. But the intuitive ability to skip a whole lot of reasoning and find a *possible* conclusion is a 267 technique of human thought that robot-makers are most anxious to imitate in their machines and programs. This talent enables humans to deal with problems that are far too complex even for a very powerful computer to tackle in any strictly logical manner.

When he seeks to imitate it, the robot-maker is choosing one of the two possible routes to 'artificial brains'. No one really has any idea how human intuition works, but it is legitimate to try to produce the same sort of talent in a machine by any means available. That is the quest for brain substitutes – machines which imitate what the brain does, rather than how it does it. It contrasts with another approach, that of inventing brain models – machines, actual or theoretical, which imitate the way the real brain works.

Substitutes for brains

Even in quite a simple game such as draughts (checkers) the player has to rely heavily on rules and strategies rather than attempt to calculate every conceivable consequence of every legitimate move. The number of possible situations, given the board and up to 24 'men', is so great that if a million computers each reviewed a million situations every second, it would take them 300 billion billion years to run through them all once. Yet twelve-year-old humans can select a sensible move in a few seconds.

In the 1950s Arthur Samuel, then with IBM, managed to program a computer with short-cuts for learning this game, so that after only ten hours' practice it began to beat him regularly. He had arranged for it to weigh up the general situation and to consider only the possible consequences of each legitimate move, for just a few moves ahead. Chess is an incomparably more complex game to analyse and although, by 1966, a computer at Stanford was playing chess against a computer in Moscow, the machines (more precisely, the programs) were admitted to be 'rather weak by human standards'.

Supposing computers could play brilliant chess, which they may well be able to do one day, should we regard them as thinkers? Almost certainly not, because we have other tests of human mental qualities. A program designed specifically to enable a computer to play chess would be useless if the machine were invited to play poker, or to help an old lady complete her income tax return. Yet we should assume that a human chess player could perform at least ordinarily well in either of these situations; if not we might regard him as an overspecialised person, a clever moron. Adaptability is characteristic of human beings; indeed we seem to be by far the most versatile of all animals.

Against this quality, too, the robot-makers have to compete. A General Problem Solver was developed by Allen Newell and Herbert Simon at the Carnegie Institute of Technology, as an early effort to program a computer to tackle a variety of problems. Using various procedures, including trial and error and working backwards from the wanted answer, the computer judged at each step whether it was getting nearer to or further from its goal. The difficulty came in translating the problem of the moment into terms suited to the general problem-solving strategy. Humans sometimes have the same sort of difficulty, as illustrated by the game shown overleaf.

The robot-makers seek to match the adaptable and not-too-logical reasoning faculties of the human mind, and to empower their machine to decide its own course of action. But reasoning needs information to work on and yet another ability of the natural brain becomes important to imitate. If the machine simply stored information just as it came in (through the artificial eye, for example) it would have a hard time recovering that information as required, even if it had a memory of sufficient capacity. The human brain analyses what the eye sees and the ear hears, and builds up a store of consistent patterns and associations – concepts and models of the outside world. That is the aim of the experiments with the teacups at Edinburgh, and similar efforts with camera 'eyes' and computers.

By the late 1960s, several of the leading groups interested in making thinking machines were all developing robots which explored the scene confronting them. At the Stanford Research Institute in California, Charles Rosen and his colleagues made a cart that carried a television camera, a rangefinder and a bumper. It roamed around a laboratory strewn like a maze with variously-shaped boxes, analysing the layout and finding a path among the boxes. Like the Edinburgh robot, it was connected by cable to a powerful computer, and its 'secret' lay in the programming.

Early hopes for the mechanisation of thought processes were too optimistic and it turns out to be quite a struggle to produce even simple manifestations of thinking in a machine. In principle, the robot-makers need the most powerful computers available, or better, to achieve anything much that resembles human thought. In practice the difficulties of writing the programs limit what can be done even with smaller computers. The aims of individual experiments are therefore limited. But the general objective still ranks among the most ambitious that men have ever set themselves.

A game made easy

The way a problem is presented, to humans or to machines, can greatly influence its difficulty. Here is a game with nine counters for two players; Donald Michie attributes it to Frank George:

① ② ③ ④ ⑤ ⑥ ⑦ ⑧ ⑨

Each player has to pick up counters by turn until one has three counters (out of more, if necessary) that add up to 15. It is really quite a difficult game. But you need never lose if you memorise the following square of numbers:

$$2 \quad 7 \quad 6$$
$$9 \quad 5 \quad 1$$
$$4 \quad 3 \quad 8$$

Every line (row, column or diagonal) adds up to 15, so that the game reduces itself to trying to complete one of the lines, and stopping the opponent from doing so. It is then strongly reminiscent of another game that looks like this:

It is the game known to some children as noughts and crosses and to others as tic-tac-toe. It is basically identical to the counters game but it is very much easier to play, because it is a visual rather than an arithmetical game.

Machines like gods

Apart from sticking to the proposition that we are now beginning to understand the mind of man in terms of brain mechanisms, I have tried up to this point to be a dispassionate reporter of some current developments in research and theory. Any conclusiveness has been due more to the scientific successes of others, than to my opinions. But that posture is not appropriate for dealing with some implications of man's current interest in the status of his mind. In the remaining pages I shall argue for tolerance and scepticism (the two sides of the liberal coin) at a time when ideology and engineering could conspire to declare man as we know him to be an obsolete slob.

Now, it is entirely possible that he is exactly that. Human civilisation may, even in our lifetime, cease its interference with the natural course of evolution. The combination of intellect and manual skill which we embody may be an aberration of nature as non-viable as many other freak species cast aside in the long history of this planet. To a few high-ranking individuals we assign the power to blow up all our cities, and to kill most of us, using the vast stockpile of H-bombs recently conjured into existence by the mind of man.

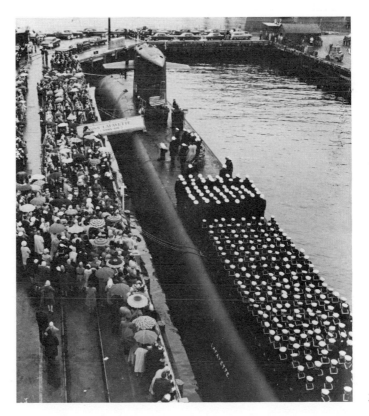

The Polaris submarine, capable of destroying sixteen cities with H-bombs, is a contemporary symbol of man's mental ability to plan the destruction of his species.

Short of Armageddon, we can go out with a whimper, in some combination of overpopulation, pollution, exhaustion of resources and civil strife. There are plenty of other species available to replace us as masters of the continents, while the future of intellect may lie in the giant brains of the handless and harmless whales. Events may easily make us obsolete, if we don't watch out.

But to suggest the voluntary liquidation of Human Nature, Inc., is quite another matter. Proposals of this kind come from diverse sources. There are some among us who hold that man is not intelligent enough and should make way for intelligent machines or supermen. Others dwell on our emotionality and aggressiveness, or on the confusion and unhappiness of our society; they would make radical changes to our mental chemistry or our upbringing as remedies for human nature.

At present, specialists in artificial intelligence would be happy if they could produce a machine ranking in intellectual capacity with an unexceptional kindergarten child. Some of them insist that they only wish to make useful new systems for industry, education and so forth. Donald Michie, for one, regrets the Frankenstein image attaching to him and his colleagues. But how are onlookers supposed to react to statements like the following, by Marvin Minsky, a pioneer of artificial intelligence at the Massachusetts Institute of Technology?

> It is unreasonable, however, to think machines could become *nearly* as intelligent as we are and then stop, or to suppose we will always be able to compete with them in wit or wisdom. Whether or not we could retain some sort of control of the machines, assuming that we would want to, the nature of our activities and aspirations would be changed utterly by the presence on earth of intellectually superior beings.

From time to time attempts are made to argue that machines comparing with, or surpassing, human beings in intelligence simply cannot be made. Sometimes they raise a point of principle. It may be the supposition that man possesses an ingredient, consciousness for example, held to be both vital for man-like intelligence and beyond the attainment of a machine. Or it may be the Gödel limit (page 263) which is said to prevent us comprehending our own minds fully – how then could we design the necessary machine? Or the argument is sometimes more practical, as it was in ending the costly failure of attempts at machine translation of language. The mechanisms of human thought may be simply far too subtle and complex to define and match on the basis of present or even foreseeable understanding. When results in artificial intelligence fall short of expectations, there are always those ready to speak of hidden obstacles standing in the way of advance.

But the available effort in artificial intelligence has so far been small in comparison with the task, which by any standards is formidable. Only continuing experiment can show whether enthusiasts are right. It would be no wiser now to deny all the possibilities of success with intelligent machines than to hold, as Victorians, that powered flight was out of the question. I think it is more useful to face the credibility of artificial intelligence and to consider why it is unthinkable that we should leave any important decisions to a super-intelligent robot.

Such abdication would amount to worship of intelligence in information-processing as the supreme or only virtue. Conventional computers are being used in ever more sophisticated

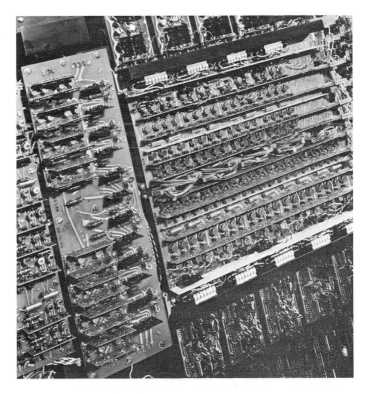

Part of the high-speed memory system of the new B 8500 computer. The world's computing power is doubling every two years or so.

ways as administrative aids up to ministerial and boardroom levels; and very useful they are too. The machines enable decisions to be made on much fuller and more up-to-date information than in the past; moreover they can carry mathematical models of the government or company operations and forecast the consequences of various possible courses of action.

273

Their limitations, though, are fairly conspicuous. There are plenty of factors in human affairs which cannot be treated mathematically except as very crude assumptions. The computer and its programs are competent only in certain kinds of problems. Overspecialisation is likely also to be a defect of foreseeable intelligent machines – unless they are made entirely man-like. In that case, the old gibe at the would-be makers of robots holds good – it's cheaper to breed them.

Horses in our heads

The old-fashioned human mind may be simply incapable of grasping some of the laws of nature, either those governing the physical universe of galaxies and atoms or those operating within the brain itself. One man who thinks that it is surprising we have understood so much already is Robert Sinsheimer, president of the American Biophysical Society. He speculates about the limits to thought inherent in the structure of the brain and how it might be extended by genetic modification. Sinsheimer is impressed by how little chemical difference there seems to be between the human genes and those of a monkey: he estimates a four-per-cent change in the chemical code of heredity since monkeys and man shared a common ancestor fifteen million years ago.

By means of further, deliberate change Sinsheimer expects that new brains can be made with sensations of undreamt intensity and of an unknown nature – a change equivalent to the introduction of colour into animal vision. Further aims might be to give the consciousness greater access to the unconscious processes of mind and to increase the amount of information it can bring to bear upon a conceptual problem. Speech, in Sinsheimer's view, is too recent an innovation for nature to have been able to perfect it, so he would like to make it faster and try to ensure that the use of words is more precise. Indeed (as he warms to his theme) why not build knowledge of a language into the brain circuits, as birds know the songs of their species?

Another approach to brain development that appeals to Sinsheimer is to seek the unusual factor in the brains of individuals of exceptional gifts, like Mozart or like Alexander Luria's memory-man S (see page 187). By such studies we shall prepare for the day when we can start pushing back the limits of our present cerebral components. He also says we should rid ourselves, along the way, of 'emotional anachronisms' like excess aggressiveness and pessimism. That seems to be a reliable way

of ensuring that, whatever freaks such a eugenic enterprise

produced, they would be judged as masterpieces by the calm and optimistic new generations.

A particularly stern critic of the present design of the human brain is Paul MacLean, of the National Institutes of Health at Bethesda, Maryland. He thinks the most striking discovery about the brain is its division into three basic cerebral units, so

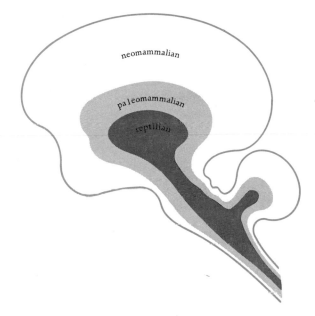

Paul MacLean's divisions of the brain led to a proposal for taming the emotional 'horse' of the middle regions of the brain.

separated by evolution and function as to lead MacLean to speak of 'schizophysiology'. The three brains of man he calls reptilian, old mammalian and new mammalian, in the style of a geologist looking at layers of rock. Indeed, they do form layers. The lowest, the reptilian brain, is essentially in the brain stem and midbrain. Above it lies the old mammalian brain, fringing the top of the brain stem, the region known as the limbic system. Surmounting it all is the new mammalian brain, newest in evolutionary terms, which in man makes up the greater part of the cerebral cortex and supplies many of his special powers.

So far so good: we have here a succinct account of the evolution of the brain. But MacLean goes on. Man's mighty new cortex is fine, he implies, but the two lower brains correspond in function to those manifest in the lower animals in which they first developed. Thus the reptilian brain, the old crocodile under our skulls, is 'a slave to precedent . . . neurosis-bound by an ancestral superego . . . inadequate machinery for learning to cope with new situations', and MacLean hints that human ritual and religion may be influenced by the reptilian counterpart in man's brain.

MacLean's sternest disapproval is saved for the old mammalian, horse-like brain. The limbic system is very much involved in emotional responses in man and monkeys (see page 58). In man, epileptic seizures in this region produce feelings of hunger, thirst, choking, terror, sadness, *déjà vu* and so on; also feelings of a paranoid nature. For MacLean, it is from this region that the 'paranoid streak in man' springs, with the sense of persecution or elation for reasons that cannot be clearly identified and for which the higher intellectual faculties invent a crazy explanation.

MacLean likens the new cortex of man to a psychiatrist trying to analyse the emotional feelings of his patient, the older brain. The essence of MacLean's idea is that our intellectual functions are carried on in the nice, new, highly-developed part of the brain, while our subjective emotions are dominated by 'a relatively crude and primitive system'. He gives sketchy technical arguments for supposing that the operational links between the new and old brains are sparse and indirect.

From MacLean's anatomy of the two camps of reason and emotion flows Arthur Koestler's proposal for a radical treatment of this human schizophysiology. He says that man – normal man – is insane. He wants to turn 'maniac into man' by the invention and distribution of a mental stabiliser, a pill which will reunite reason and emotion and restore the 'hierarchic order', by which he means the submission of emotion to reason.

The MacLean-Koestler view of man is picturesque and appealing in the way that all fables are appealing. Curiously enough, one of MacLean's most recent accounts of his idea of the three brains appears in a book edited by Arthur Koestler (with John Smythies) called *Beyond Reductionism*. But the scheme is reductionism with a vengeance. It alleges that a large part of human conduct, the emotional side, can be explained as elementary responses shown by lower animals. The proposal that we should all mend ourselves with a molecule, in the form of a drug, is a denial of the complexity of our minds and motives.

Reason and emotion

Even if Koestler's rationality pill were practicable, despite the known shortcomings of mind-control measures, the diagnosis is very dubious indeed. If the old horse in the human head is supposed to be an animal of pure, unbridled emotion, why are horses so much less emotional than humans, letting us, literally, put bridles on them? It is the more complex brain, with most of that complexity in the neomammalian cortex, which is

more emotional.

Although the limbic system (the 'horse') is undoubtedly an engine of emotion, the new cortex amplifies the intensity and effects of emotion, using the very connections which MacLean minimises. The claims of schizophysiology are in any case severely dented by the accomplishments of Anand's yogi and Neal Miller's rats and patients, in controlling not just the lower regions of the brain, but the most horse-like and crocodile-like internal functions of the body.

The tradition of western philosophy that reason is good and emotion is bad is still very persistent and 'invidious', to use Miller's epithet. It continues despite all the evidence that uncurbed reason can destroy civilisation with computer-guided H-bombs, for esoteric purposes of policy, in a way that the most homicidal rage of an individual could not begin to

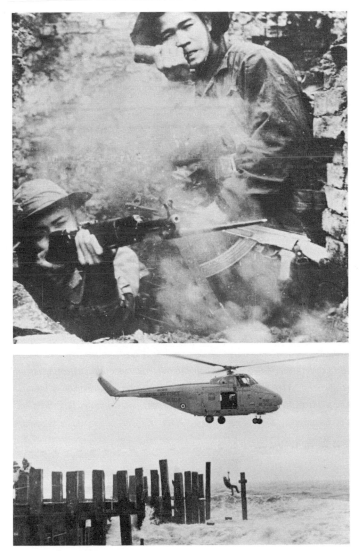

The mind of man can devote itself with equal zeal to taking life or saving life. Right: Vietcong infantrymen at Quang Tri. Below: a desperate bid to rescue a man trapped behind the groyne in a rising tide, at Lowestoft.

match. The confusion arises because we say 'reason' when we mean 'reasonableness' – which implies a lot of love and altruism as well as logic – while we talk of emotion as if it were all blind rage. Yet the mechanisms of arousal and emotional disturbance are cardinal to all activity; even a Socrates would not bother to reason unless motivated to do so.

If the human balance of reason and emotion were not pretty good we could not have prospered as we have. The success of most humans at most times in sustaining the right emotional tone for everyday life, lapsing neither into apathy nor into fanaticism, is surely impressive. The upgrading of the emotions by the new discoveries of Anand and Miller, concerning the voluntary control of the glands and bodily organs, should change the valuation as the message sinks in. It is no longer even legitimate to call emotion 'irrational', if by that is meant a dissociation from the workings of the cerebral cortex.

The bodily responses that give physical expression and intensification of emotion can be learnt in the ordinary way. At least some of the differences in temperament between individuals may be due to differences in their upbringing. Differences in emotional habits from one nation or culture to another may be to that extent self-sustaining and based upon learned physical responses within the autonomic nervous system. Miller gives the example of Homer's world, in which adult heroes so often 'let the big tears fall'. Reflection on the discovery of the voluntary control of the autonomic nervous system may, in the years ahead, show it to be the key to much fresh understanding of human nature.

The effects of childhood experience upon adult personality are known to be real but they are vaguely specified and often unpredictable. The same unpleasant event may haunt one person for life and leave another unscathed. These differences may make much more sense if they are relatable to the excitability or vulnerability of particular glands and organs. When new links are traced between mind and body, expressions such as 'stony-hearted', 'warm-blooded', 'gutless' and the like may no longer seem quite so fanciful as they have done to recent medicine. In any case, the scope for modifying our treatment of other people, to improve our communal lives, is probably very great. How far are we prepared to go, in doing it systematically?

Skinner's utopia

B. F. Skinner is a man of many accomplishments. He established a new branch of experimental psychology and pioneered teaching machines. He trained pigeons to be suicide pilots in gliding bombs – a project which, unlike the Russian use of dogs to blow up tanks, did not bear fruit before the end of the war in 1945. But Skinner reckons that one of the most important things he ever did was to write a novel and he is happy to display the exponential curve of its sales, now soaring more than twenty years after its first publication.

Walden Two is a utopia of the classical form: a fictional account of a visit to an isolated community where life is very different from what we know. Behind the rural, cultured serenity of Walden Two is behavioural engineering, the application of the techniques of psychological conditioning to social life, as explained by the founder of the community:

> No, Mr Castle, when a science of behaviour has once been achieved, there's no alternative to a planned society. We can't leave mankind to an accidental or biased control. But by using the principle of positive reinforcement – carefully avoiding force or the threat of force – we can preserve a personal sense of freedom.

A group of Planners and Managers runs Walden Two. The novel eloquently puts the case for limited despotism against the 'pious fraud' of democracy in the untidy, accidental, unhappy world outside Walden Two. The long-term aim is the design of personalities.

'Give me the specification and I'll give you the man.' Skinner is apt to quote his novel's hero, Frazier, as other scholars cite authorities in their field. This particular remark once prompted George Wald, a Harvard biologist, publicly to retort: 'Not if I can shoot you first.' Skinner is well accustomed to such anger about his ideas. He persists in believing in Walden Two and he says that, two decades later, he would make only small changes – for example, in paying more attention to crime. Unlike his very bold predecessor, John B. Watson, who offered to make a doctor or an artist out of any child, Skinner allows for differences in IQ; but he insists that behaviour can be shaped, to make a better world.

The practical difficulties of shaping humans in the mass may be greater than Skinner supposes, even if done voluntarily, as he thinks it will be. Yet Skinner relates his ideas to the Christian ethic and to the brotherhood of man. Opposing them on principle makes one feel a little like a *laissez-faire* reactionary and a friend of iniquity, chaos and strife. Neglecting Skinner's ideas would be to ignore one of the clearest restatements of ideal communism since St Thomas More's *Utopia*; it would also overlook the likelihood that people will try to apply behavioural engineering, for good or evil purposes.

Skinner's comes closer to current politics than do the schemes for superseding present-day man by intelligent machines or with *sapiens plus*. Here is no plan for altering man by genetic engineering or drugs, but it declares us obsolete in other ways. Why is it to be rejected?

The persistent reasons are present ignorance and the merits of diversity. No one has the knowledge or the right to say what human beings should be like, beyond the ephemeral and collective dictates of social mores, economic realities and the criminal law. And even if someone did know exactly what was ideal for our present circumstances, the production of ideal people would consume all our alternative futures in the cold fire of contentment and mutual approval. Saying so is not a defence of 'good old human fallibility' but an attack upon it, as embodied in the would-be Planners and Managers.

A matter of time

When we distinguish the 'human' from the 'animal' or 'bestial', we usually mean reasonable conduct and the display of the kindlier emotions. But the uniqueness of man, compared with other animals, is not so simple. Being inherently more emotional, he achieves civilised conduct by prolonged learning. His unusual reasoning ability, skills of hand and powers of language modify his emotional behaviour. Animals can know nothing of romantic love or the legalised murder of warfare. In the latter case, it is reason rather than animal-like emotion that produces the peculiarly dangerous conduct. Mild, impersonal feelings of aggression towards another people are immensely amplified by the jargon of nationalism and the intellectual skills of the weapon-makers.

And what distinguishes man from any artificial mind he might make, a super-intelligent computer or a superman? When we say 'human', as opposed to 'mechanical' or 'technical', we usually imply feelings and emotion. Arranging that a computer should exhibit emotional responses or disturbances, resembling the human ones, is not at all difficult, but they are fakes. The big difference in this, as in other respects, is that the human characteristics have evolved and developed. It is above all a matter of time. If the formidable task were undertaken of making a robot exactly like a man, the product would presumably act approximately like a man. But the engineers would, of course, be cribbing the designs of nature. Any omission or addition to the cerebral circuits would be liable to upset a very fine balance; even minor variations, such as a change in the speed of transmission of nerve signals, would have unpredictable consequences. But even if all that were taken care of, an automaton would not be human without also being programmed to grow inside a womb and to experience all the joys, fears and lessons of childhood – unless, with immense ingenuity, the engineers gave their machine an artificial but realistic biography written into the brain.

As two kinds of designers are being compared, it may be permissable to personify Mother Nature for a moment. She has no goal, no prejudice for or against intellect; she is not even greatly concerned with efficient use of energy and raw materials by living systems. She has only one test – viability in the complex environment of the planet. Every basic system of the human body has been thoroughly tested, from the enzymes that extract energy from sugar and oxygen to the ways of coding logical operations in brain tissue. Even our emotional and social problems are not especially novel to Mother Nature: she has experimented for millions of years with social life in many species of animals, juggling self-interest with the benefits of communal action. We, the brash, self-confident inheritors of all this expertise may have appreciated, so far, only one per cent or less of the factors taken care of in our genetic design.

Like other products of nature, the mind of man, in its turn, has been tested under the most diverse conditions imaginable, from the gamelands of Africa to the surface of the moon; it has

The human brain enters another environment. Imperfect though our minds may be, they show no signs of exhausting their capacity for achievement. Some commentators suggest, on the contrary, that we shall have to put a brake on our creativity.

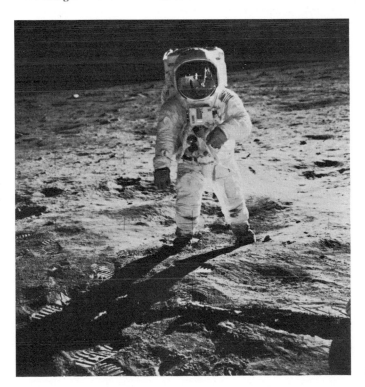

coolly faced tasks ranging from the outwitting of whales to the decipherment of Minoan script; it has shown itself capable of self-sacrifice in desperate circumstances and of restless creative energy when affluent conditions might make it lazy. It has conceived cathedrals and parliaments, open-heart surgery and zip-fasteners. For what else it may prove competent in the centuries ahead, no one can guess.

It would be fatuous to suggest that man is biologically perfect, in a cosmic sense. Any reading of history, or observation of our present follies and wickedness, or speculation about what species may evolve in the next billion years, should dispel such conceit. But it is equally fatuous to suppose that anyone alive today can specify in what respect we are deficient, seeing that both our judgement and our basic human nature are so overlaid with ephemeral ways of life, interests, ideologies and ignorance. Of course human aggressiveness is deadly dangerous in our present world, but who dares to promise that ablation of our capacity for anger, righteous or unrighteous, would not be potentially as dehumanising as the loss of love?

Roughly speaking, we have to take humans as we find them and adapt our societies to man rather than man to society. Of course, 'as we find them' begs all the nature-nurture questions about the effects on the mind of upbringing and local cultures. The very different kinds of society that will emerge during the next few generations will make people somewhat different, just as we differ in our mental furnishings from our stone-age forefathers. But some durable traits, including aggressiveness, probably have to be canalised and counterbalanced rather than ignored or repressed.

The escape from certainty

Humans are obliged to compile simplified models and working hypotheses of the world around them, in their brains, if they are to make any sense of their environment. The elementary mechanisms of vision and hearing make this policy unavoidable. As we saw early on (page 59), emotional effects can distort the facts of the world and set us on the high road to prejudice. Otto Klineberg, of the Centre for the Study of Intergroup Relations in Paris, has specified some of the mechanisms that reinforce an established prejudice. He is dealing particularly with ethnic and national prejudice, but the same processes are relevant to judgements in science, the arts and public policy:

1. *Selective inattention* (noticing only what fits with our prejudices, ignoring what does not).

2. *Distortion of imagery* (misperceiving what we cannot avoid attending to).
3. *Making exceptions* (shrugging off as atypical what we cannot misperceive).
4. *Reinterpretation* (choosing from alternative ways of looking at the self-same facts – 'I am a brave commando; he is a fanatical terrorist').

Compound with these (as Klineberg does) the various unconscious mechanisms that influence our thought processes and you have powerful reasons why human judgement is often to be mistrusted. But eradicating prejudice entirely from ordinary mental life is probably as impossible as writing a novel without words. Even a superman or a super-computer would need its practical working assumptions, based upon inadequate evidence and its built-in defences against loss of self-confidence. Among humans some durable personal prejudices in favour of wife and friends, for example, are always respected. On particular issues, such as race or superstition, careful research and argument can help to mitigate and erode prejudice. But Jerome Bruner of Harvard suspects that 'neurological editing' makes ideal scientific objectivity unattainable.

Natural science exhibits a characteristic human aim – the urge to simplify, to comprehend an elephant as a bundle of chemicals, to sum up the laws of the universe in a dozen mathematical equations or, better still, in one. It has been a successful policy in arriving at principles of cosmic forces, natural selection and molecular genetics which a schoolboy can grasp. Scientists rescue themselves from the inevitable absurdities fairly quickly by their obligatory regard for verification and criticism; the intellectual health of science is the least of our present worries. Of greater concern is the similar urge of the human intellect to make grand simplifications in public affairs.

The quest for simplicity may not pay off in the study of systems which are inherently and necessarily complex: the interaction between species and the natural environment, or that very special interactor, the human mind. The laws governing the mind can hardly be as simple as those governing atoms. As human society is an assembly of minds, it is even more optimistic to suppose that its mechanisms are within our ready comprehension, or discoverable in a cursory reading of history.

But when you believe in the supreme virtue of your own nation, race or party, or in the infallibility of your leader whether he be the Pope or Mao Tse-Tung, how much less

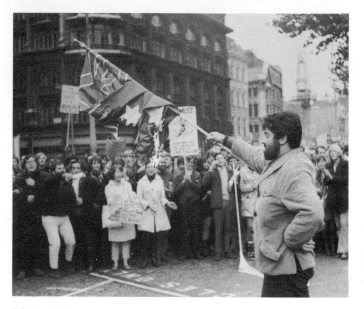

Symbolism is turned against itself. The national flag is a mark, not just of organisation by states, but of the human quest for simple embodiments of virtue in an extremely complex world.

confusing the world becomes! The evidence of human susceptibility to prejudice suggests that any absolute belief is liable to be a pathological distortion of perception (including, of course, any absolute belief that all faiths or strong convictions are necessarily false). And nothing could be more absolute than a proposal for remaking or replacing man.

To alter ourselves to fit the Procrustean bed of twentieth-century society is absurd, especially as this society is plainly obsolescent. We are rapidly moving towards an automated economy in which people will be paid to do nothing and in which computers will execute much of the middle range of 'intellectual' and skilled work for which youngsters are now schooled as industrial cannon-fodder. With the economic problems of ten thousand years largely solved, the opportunities for the transformation of society to suit human nature will be almost unlimited. There will be no pressing need to regard IQ or military skill or any of the historically admired virtues as socially desirable.

Even creativity may be down-rated before long, in public affairs. That is the forecast of a Japanese psychologist, Masanao Toda of Hokkaido University. At an international congress in London in 1969 he suggested that future generations would look back on us with envy, as privileged participants in a 'carnival of mankind'. We have freedom of creative action but our social systems are breaking down under the strain of absorbing its consequences. The present era of great change must soon, in Toda's view, give way to a nearly steady state, with a fluid and self-disciplined society deliberately designed to dissipate creative energy. Potential 'troublemakers' will be assigned extremely difficult tasks, like assembling a new planet out of the asteroids, or teaching animals to talk.

There is resonance here with Herbert Marcuse, the would-be reconciler of Marx and Freud, who has been admired by some of the students in revolt around the world. Whatever the provenance and consequences of Marcuse's theories, there may be sense in his suggestion that the time is coming when man 'surveys what has been achieved through centuries of misery and hecatombs of victims, and decides that it is enough, and that it is time to enjoy what he has'.

My own proposal (*The Environment Game*) was that *Homo sapiens* should recognise both his origins as a hunter and the terrible damage he has done to the planet as farmer; he should turn gamekeeper and devote his energies to restoring and enjoying the natural environment. All such prescriptions are fragmentary, but at least they suggest how life in the twenty-first century may be utterly different from ours. An obvious reason, though, why mankind is not quite ready to rest on its laurels is that many people in the world continue in their ancient misery and have precious little to enjoy.

Nor can mankind, in political turmoil, wait with perfect patience for the advancement of our understanding of the brain. But the growing sense of biological and intellectual complexity and the abandonment of simple principles, now apparent among brain researchers, are not badly matched to other trends in human thinking. As the artists discovered a generation or two before the technocrats and the student rebels, the western world at least has entered an age of doubt. Gone are the divine sanction of religion, the self-confidence of empire and the assurance of tidy political or economic theory, whether revolutionary or reactionary. Even technological advance is no longer regarded as self-evidently desirable. Nothing is that simple any more.

This realisation may be the beginning of wisdom. In the head of each one of us there is continual interplay between the need to reflect and the need to act. We have probably overvalued action and its attendant excitement. If we wish to tame ourselves before the H-bombs fill the sky with fire, our collective policies must, first and last, give scope for reflection. What the new awareness of the immense complexity of human ecology, of the human mind and of human ambitions makes obsolete is not man but his slogans – excepting perhaps that of Oliver Cromwell, who was no woolly-minded liberal: 'I beseech you, in the bowels of Christ, think it possible you may be mistaken.'

Index